White Drug Cultures and Regulation in London, 1916–1960

Christopher Hallam

White Drug Cultures and Regulation in London, 1916–1960

palgrave
macmillan

Christopher Hallam
Global Drug Policy Observatory
Swansea University
Swansea, UK

ISBN 978-3-030-06913-1 ISBN 978-3-319-94770-9 (eBook)
https://doi.org/10.1007/978-3-319-94770-9

Softcover re-print of the Hardcover 1st edition 2018

Printed on acid-free paper

This Palgrave Macmillan imprint is published by the registered company Springer Nature Switzerland AG
The registered company address is: Gewerbestrasse 11, 6330 Cham, Switzerland

Acknowledgements

This book is based upon PhD research carried out at the London School of Hygiene and Tropical Medicine. My thanks and appreciation go to my research supervisor, Professor Virginia Berridge, who guided me patiently and with good humour through the long research process and taught me to think like a historian.

My advisory committee, consisting of Professor Susanne MacGregor and Dr Alex Mold, provided valuable encouragement and advice.

Dr Stuart Anderson supplied me with a lucid account of the more technical relationships obtaining between the legislation and regulatory systems covering dangerous drugs and poisons.

Pamela Ford, the archive manager at the Royal College of Physicians, was particularly helpful in unearthing the minutes of the 1938 Committee on Drug Addiction.

The staff at the National Archives were patient with my frequent requests for assistance and helped me access an apparently inexhaustible knowledge base.

A sizeable group of individuals were kind enough to permit me to draw on their expertise. They included Professor Dave Bewley Taylor, Professor Jim Mills, the Rev. Ken Leech, Marek Kohn, Philip Hoare and Philip Bottomley. Numerous others contributed in one way or another, as discussants, archivists, librarians, printers, baristas; and while most must remain nameless, my gratitude for their services endures.

Molly Beck and Oliver Dyer at Palgrave Macmillan guided me smoothly through the process of publication.

Finally, thanks go to my wife Michelle, daughter Gabriela and grandchildren Eva and Lucas, respectively, nine and six years old at the time of writing, who regularly came to inhabit my study, spinning on my chair and stealing my pens while I toiled at my desk. The book is dedicated to them.

Contents

CHAPTER 1

Introduction

Introduction: The Quiet Times

The quiet times. This was the term given by British civil servant and student of drug regulation, Bing Spear, who worked at the Home Office Drugs Branch between 1952 and 1986. The period reaching from the late 1920s to the early 1960s was regarded as 'quiet' because it was believed, by Spear and by the majority of the academic researchers, that there was little or no 'drug underground' in these years and that those dependent on morphine or heroin were middle-aged, middle-class addicts who complied with the medical model and with the doctors that supplied them. This book explores the quiet times, and just how quiet they really were.

For much of the twentieth century, a kind of dance was played out between the forces that sought to regulate what were then known as 'dangerous drugs', restricting their use to 'medical and scientific' purposes, and those who wished to consume these substances for pleasure and entertainment. This book maps out the movements of this dance during the half-century of the classic 'British System', a period that has hitherto been explored by historians only at its extremities, its beginning and its end. The book takes two interwoven analytical targets—the white drug culture and the web of regulation that was brought to bear upon it. Most histories of drugs have concentrated either on the regulation of drugs or on transgressive populations and drug cultures; a key argument here is that the two are mutually constitutive and best explored together.

C. Hallam, *White Drug Cultures and Regulation in London, 1916–1960*, https://doi.org/10.1007/978-3-319-94770-9_1

The book examines the emergence, development and operation of the white drug culture in Britain—particularly London—together with its regulatory architecture. It contends that current views situating the advent of the opioid culture in the 1950s and 1960s are based on a number of erroneous assumptions and readings and that a heroin- or morphine- and cocaine- using culture ('white drugs') emerged during the interwar period. The 1930s, in particular, saw this culture crystallising out of upper-class bohemia and from the night-time economy of London's West End. In addition, the role played by the prescribing doctors of the 'British System' was a key component in this formative process.

What became known and mythologised as 'the British System' was designed to regulate the use of those materials that were then termed 'dangerous drugs'. In this work, I understand the latter term as referring not so much to a pharmacological and pharmaceutical object as a *cultural* one—a symbolic object that was, and still is, deployed as an indicator of the health or pathology of individuals and societies. At least as much as they are chemicals, drugs are objects of social and cultural war.[1] The UK's system of dealing with the consumption of these substances, which often involved the medical supply of doses to their consumers, came to be known as the 'British System', particularly in the USA, which, in its domestic setting, developed a highly restrictive set of arrangements centred on the prohibition of heroin.

The Rolleston Committee and the British System

The 1920 Dangerous Drugs Act was established in order to satisfy the obligations to which Britain had signed up when it ratified the International Opium Convention of 1912.[2] While minimal regulations had previously applied to drugs such as opium, cocaine and morphine, these substances could now only be produced, exchanged and consumed by those authorised by the Act, or by individuals possessing a valid prescription from a

[1] J. Derrida (1989) 'The Rhetoric of Drugs' in Alexander, A. & Roberts, M. S. (eds.) *High Culture: reflections on addiction and modernity* (Albany: State University of New York Press, 1989) pp. 19–42.

[2] P. Bean, *The Social Control of Drugs* (London: Martin Robertson, 1974) p. 23. See also W. B. McAllister, *Drug Diplomacy in the Twentieth Century: An international history* (London and New York: Routledge, 2000) pp. 9–39.

medical practitioner.[3] The objective was to confine such 'dangerous drugs' to 'medical and legitimate purposes', an imperative deriving from the International Opium Convention.[4] However, though robust policing did succeed in limiting drug use and largely suppressing the street drug trade in London's West End, the problem of the doctor as gatekeeper to drugs, and of the forging of prescriptions, continued to grow. For the Home Office, which was the government department responsible for regulating dangerous drugs, the core problem was the prescription of drugs to addicts by doctors, which it sought to curtail, particularly in cases of long-term or indefinite supply, and which it regarded as merely pandering to the drug habit rather than constituting a bona fide medical treatment.

In response to these conditions, a committee was set up under the chairmanship of the eminent physician Humphrey Rolleston, its primary brief being to consider in what circumstances, if any, 'the supply of morphine and heroin…to persons suffering from addiction to those drugs may be regarded as medically advisable'.[5] The conclusions of the Rolleston Committee with respect to this question form the core of what became known as the 'British System'. Owing to their subsequent importance, these passages are worth quoting in full:

> There are two groups of persons suffering from addiction to whom administration of morphine or heroin may be regarded as legitimate medical treatment namely:
>
> (a) Those who are undergoing treatment for cure of the addiction by the gradual withdrawal method;
>
> (b) Persons for whom, after every effort has been made for the cure of the addiction, the drug cannot be completely withdrawn, either because: (i) Complete withdrawal produces serious symptoms which cannot be satisfactorily treated under the ordinary conditions of private practice; or (ii) The patient, while capable of leading a useful and fairly normal

[3] Prior to this, the Defence of the Realm Act regulation 40b (DORA 40b) was in place. Introduced in 1916 amidst fears of mass cocaine use amongst servicemen, it imposed similar restrictions on opium and cocaine. See V. Berridge, 'War conditions and narcotics control: the passing of the Defence of the Realm Act regulation 40B' *Journal of Social Policy*, 7, (1978) pp. 285–304.

[4] International Opium Convention of 1912 (The 'Hague Convention'), Article 9. *The American Journal of International Law*, 6 (3) Supplement: Official Documents, (1912), pp. 177–192.

[5] *Departmental Committee on Morphine and Heroin Addiction: Report* (London: HMSO, 1926). Minutes of Appointment.

> life so long as he takes a certain non-progressive quantity, usually small, of the drug of addiction, ceases to be able to do so when the regular allowance is withdrawn.[6]

The British System, then, was understood as an institutional and therapeutic regime that viewed addiction as a disease and sought to treat it by permitting doctors to supply legitimate doses of drugs, usually on prescription, though doctors could also directly supply doses to their addict patients by injection. The system was established by the regulatory take-up of Rolleston's recommendations. While the concept of the British System has received extensive critical comment from UK researchers sceptical toward the claims of American liberals, it is worth recalling that the Rolleston Committee's report was a highly significant text, and had considerable impact on the lives of those dependent on the drugs in question, whose counterparts in the USA did indeed suffer greatly at the hands of prohibitive laws.[7] That said, the notion of the British System has resulted in considerable distortion and led to some significant lacunae in research.[8] The system of regulation in place in the classic years of British drug control included, in an integral role, the Home Office, the police and the courts; it was never an exclusively medical approach. Moreover, the practices of 'drug treatment' themselves involved the exercise of power over the mind and body of the addict; the 'treatment or control' dichotomy is a misleading formulation.[9]

Exploring the Quiet Times

The customary story of illicit drug use in Britain tells us that following its initial blooming during and immediately after the First World War, the authorities were successful in the suppression of this early drug culture,

[6] Ibid. Conclusions and Recommendations. n.p.

[7] One UK critic termed the British System '(a) system of masterly inactivity in the face of a non-existent problem…' D. Downes, *Contrasts in Tolerance: Post War Penal Policy in the Netherlands and in England and Wales* (Oxford: Clarendon Press, 1993) p. 89.

[8] For a consideration of the British System, see V. Berridge, 'The British System and its history: myth and reality' in J. Strang and M. Gossop (eds) *Heroin Addiction and the British System: Volume 1: Origins and Evolution* (London and New York: Routledge, 2005). G. Pearson, 'Drug-Control Policies in Britain', *Crime and Justice*, 14 (1991) pp. 167–227.

[9] A. Mold *Heroin: The Treatment of Addiction in Twentieth Century Britain* (DeKalb, Illinois: Northern Illinois University Press, 2008).

leaving opiate use confined to a respectable and compliant population of middle-class, medicalised addicts. Many academic drug historians gained the impression that there was, essentially, little or nothing to study during this period, the narcotic landscape being more or less bare. The use of drugs for pleasure, the story goes, did not arise until the postwar boom of the 1960s, when a new type of consumer arrived on the scene—young, working class, male, and susceptible to the pernicious influence of the discourse of the North American 'junkie'. The intervening period between the 1920s and the late 1950s has been termed the 'quiet times'.[10]

As far back as the 1930s, Alfred Lindesmith, a politically engaged US sociologist who received graduate training at the University of Chicago, was arguing that the UK lacked a drug culture as a result of the country's medical orientation toward drug control. Lindesmith was a continuous thorn in the side of the US control system, whose punitive ethos he strongly opposed; he was allegedly subjected to a smear campaign by Harry Anslinger, chief of the Federal Bureau of Narcotics, intended to suppress his dissident views on the US approach.[11] Lindesmith was an early proponent of the British System, believing that the prescription of opiates to addicts had, among other things, prevented the formation of a drug culture. It became a widespread view among supporters of the British System and those who had been influenced by them.[12]

Of course, the narrative of the quiet times was not the only reason why this gap has remained in the historiography. The specific political focus of many UK sociologists and the social and cultural changes associated with the Second World War directed research into drug-using groups toward postwar working-class youth culture. In addition, the numbers involved in using drugs for pleasure and entertainment *were* small during the quiet times, even if the Home Office's data, which were drawn from often highly ineffective police inspections of retail pharmacies, almost certainly under-represented the size of the drug-using population. Whatever the precise

[10] H. B. Spear, 'The early years of Britain's drug situation in practice: up to the 1960s' in J. Strang and M. Gossop, (eds) *Heroin Addiction and the British System: Volume 1: Origins and Evolution* (London and New York: Routledge, 2005) p. 20.

[11] J. F. Galliher, D. P. Keys, M. Elsner, 'Lindesmith v. Anslinger: An Early Government Victory in the Failed War on Drugs.' *The Journal of Criminal Law and Criminology*, 88, (1998) pp. 661–682.

[12] E. M. Schur, *Narcotic Addiction in Britain and America: The Impact of Public Policy* (London: Tavistock, 1963); and: A. S. Trebach *The Heroin Solution* Second Edition (Bloomington, Indiana: Unlimited Publishing, 2006).

figures were—and they are lost to us now—the period's opioid users possessed a cultural significance out of proportion with their numbers. Furthermore, a detailed examination of the historical records indicates that they did form a distinct drug culture, mostly centred on London.

Sources

There is precious little academic historical work on the drug-using networks of the quiet times, nor on the regulatory regime designed to prevent them from using drugs for nonmedical purposes. Such research as does exist is reviewed in this chapter. However, the primary sources upon which the project depends are archival ones, located in the National Archive, the British Library, the Royal College of Physicians Archive and various online newspaper archives.

Perhaps the most important of these materials consist in Home Office, Metropolitan Police and Ministry of Health files on the regulation of the drug cultures of the 1930s. One of these, dealing with the Chelsea-based addict Brenda Dean Paul, is a large and extremely rich source. It was opened under a Freedom of Information Act request by the author, as were several other files dealing with the doctors who prescribed for these and other groups of addicts. Another source that would have been of immense value to researchers was the Addicts Index, a listing officially begun in 1934 but which had probably been kept from the mid-1920s, in order to monitor the prevalence of addiction in the UK. To the great loss of historical research on drug use in the UK, the Addicts Index was mistakenly destroyed in the 1990s and its data lost.[13] This makes it impossible to undertake a detailed critical examination of the way the Index was compiled and cases assigned to its various categories. Historical data on addiction remain, consequently, largely speculative, though Home Office officials have readily acknowledged the insecure foundations on which the statistics rested.

A second set of sources upon which I have drawn extensively, and one that complements the official state documentation, is that of newspaper reports and articles from the period. The advent of the World Wide Web has facilitated an extensive new field of newspaper and magazine resources for the use of the historical researcher. Those consulted included British

[13] This information was gleaned from personal discussions with a former member of the Home Office staff.

national daily newspapers, international newspapers from the USA and Asia and regional and local UK news publications. During preliminary methodological discussions of the project, I found that a number of my interlocutors regarded newspapers as 'unreliable' and unsafe to use. However, I did not employ these publications as arbiters of historical accuracy; rather, they provided otherwise unobtainable biographical, sartorial and other personal details, as well as contained social and cultural understandings that speak to the contemporary landscape inhabited by these groups and individuals. As Adrian Bingham has observed, for the public of the 1930s, 'the national daily newspaper was perhaps the most important channel of information about contemporary life'.[14] This was likely to be especially true in the case of nonmedical drug use, of which many people had no direct experience.

One further source of which I have made use but is too diverse and wide-ranging to review here is the mosaic of biography, memoir, letters, diaries and other accounts generated by those whose lives were lived amidst the bohemias, smart sets, modernisms and criminal milieux whose paths crossed in the social landscape of interwar and early postwar London. Many of these works contain relatively little which is of use to the drug researcher—until one stumbles onto a new character, a hitherto unsuspected connection between groups, a previously unknown nightclub, a street corner where customers awaited suppliers. These texts range from the ghost-written biography of a drug user, which turns out to be assembled from the barely informed opinions of a journalist, to a contemporary guidebook on eating out in 1930s London.

A Short Note Regarding Theoretical Approach

The theoretical approach employed in this work is an eclectic and pragmatic one, and this approach is tightly interwoven with its methodological choices. The research pays considerable attention to the individuals involved in the events and processes explored. This is because in the formation of the subculture studied here, the parts played by specific people are crucial; for instance, without Brenda Dean Paul's 'persuasively poised example', the opioid culture that crystallised out of upper-class bohemian Chelsea in the late 1920s and early 1930s would not have emerged as it

[14] A. Bingham, *Gender, Modernity and the Popular Press in Interwar Britain* (Oxford: Oxford University Press, 2004) p. 3.

did.[15] I do not mean to propose that without this individual the subculture would not have formed at all, only that it would have been different. The point is that these kinds of historical processes depend on particular people, in specific times and places, and that those involved are not merely the bearers of vast impersonal processes, or historical units which are fully interchangeable. Consequently, what is required to trace the trajectory of such events is what one might call a kind of network biography. At the same time, I seek to trace in the fabric of their lives the impacts of forces that are indeed vast and impersonal, such as the growth of the state and the regulation of the medical profession.

Beyond these few considerations, I will conclude this short discussion by reference to Frank Mort's description of the position adopted in his *Capital Affairs*, which, he explains, 'adopts a middle ground position between…cultural power understood discursively and structurally and a more humanistic understanding of history propelled by egocentric actors and directed social movements'.[16] This summarises neatly the position taken here. I will now proceed to a detailed review of the key literatures utilised in building the framework within which the research materials are analysed.

The Use of Hebdige's 'Subculture'

While British sociologist Dick Hebdige used ideas from structuralism to analyse youth subcultures from the postwar period, I will argue that the conceptual tools he provided—which do not oblige us to commit to any general theoretical framework—are extremely useful and relevant to understanding the cultural exchanges surrounding the networks explored by the present project. Hebdige conceptualised subcultures as groups which disrupt social codes through styles of clothing, speech and conduct. Objects are absorbed into different, subcultural fields of meaning; for example, when taken out of the hands of the (male) doctor where, according to the dominant culture, it 'belongs', the hypodermic syringe becomes a sign of disorder in the clutches of an unruly young woman. Hebdige contends that, for all the outrage and alarm that surrounds

[15] F. Wyndham, *Mrs Henderson* (New York: Moyer Bell, 1985) p. 60. See page 73 of the present text for a fuller discussion.

[16] F. Mort, *Capital Affairs: London and the Making of the Permissive Society* (London: Yale University Press, 2010) pp. 10–11.

them, subcultures are 'just so much graffiti on a prison wall'; that is, they are confined to the symbolic realm, and cannot bring about the large-scale changes sought by the political left to which Hebdige subscribed. Nonetheless, they are, he suggests, culturally and socially significant. As noted by the critic D. J. Taylor in relation to the actions of the 'bright young people' (BYP) of the 1920s and 1930s: 'These were, on the face of it, modest rebellions – minor adjustments to conventional behaviour, a revolt symbolised by short skirts, high heels and cigarette cases – yet their effect on large sections of upper-class society was profoundly unsettling.'[17] Those who formed an opiate subculture out of this 'smart bohemian' set found that their unsettling effect was not limited to the upper classes and was *much* more disturbing. Hebdige's tools, therefore, are very useful in analysing the 'modest rebellions', the transgression of social and cultural codes accomplished by the early drug cultures, and in understanding why such numerically tiny groups caused such anxieties and alarms amongst those who regarded the contemporary code of meanings and relationships as representing the natural order of things.

There are debates concerning the validity and usefulness—or otherwise—of the terms 'cultures' and 'subcultures'. I intend to pass these by, since both of have uses and their pitfalls. 'Drug culture', 'drug subculture', 'drug scene' and 'underground' are used more or less interchangeably in this work, since their meaning is either clear already or will be become so upon acquaintance with the materials encountered in reading this book.

Sexual Subcultures and Drugs

Another body of literature on which my research has drawn is that of the history of sexuality. The work of Foucault has been seminal here, de-essentialising sexuality and opening it up to cultural analysis.[18] Countless authors have moved into the general territory that Foucault marked out, though few of these have engaged with the history of drugs and addiction. This is surprising, since the urban and metropolitan settings in which marginalised sexualities flourished in the nineteenth and twentieth centuries

[17] D. J. Taylor, *Bright Young People: The Rise and Fall of a Generation: 1918–1940* (London: Chatto and Windus, 2007) p. 45. The bright young people are discussed in Chap. 3.

[18] M. Foucault, *The Will to Knowledge: The History of Sexuality Volume 1* (London: Penguin Books, 1998).

have mapped closely onto those in which drug subcultures emerged. As Sadie Plant has observed: 'Sex and drugs are both entangled in…spirals of power and resistance, regulation and escape…(producing) a new underground with its own signs and secret gestures, cryptic messages, dress codes, glances, clubs, street corners…Cities contained new maps, geography of stolen pleasures, a new commerce of desire….'[19] Similarly, Susan Zieger points out that homosexuality and addiction shared an embedding in narratives of deviance, and were to be found together in outcast urban districts along with the sex industry, gambling and dubious nightclubs.[20] Few historians have followed in the footsteps of cultural studies onto these territories, excepting, as we have seen, Berridge and Kohn. More recently, Caroline Acker has demonstrated the shaping of 'the American junkie' in the Progressive Era campaigns against vice and the zones in which it had taken root.[21] However, the intimate relationships obtaining in the UK between subcultures of sexuality and drugs await detailed historical investigation. In Matt Houlbrook's excellent study of *Queer London*, the superimposition one upon another in metropolitan geography of the haunts of queer subculture (on which Houlbrook concentrates) and that of illicit drugs is striking and reflected the close overlapping of the respective networks.[22] I shall explore this geographical and subcultural overlap further in the chapters that follow.

The literatures discussed in the foregoing passages provide a background for the emerging white drug subculture, and the regulatory discourses and practices that were deployed in an attempt at controlling it. This introduction situates the first white drug subcultures to appear in Britain in the 'quiet times' of the interwar years, which have previously

[19] S. Plant, *Writing on Drugs* (London: Faber and Faber, 1999) p. 154.

[20] S. Zieger, *Inventing the Addict: Drugs, Race and Sexuality in Nineteenth Century British and American Literature* (Amherst: University of Massachusetts, 2008) p. 159.

[21] C. Acker, *Creating the American Junkie: Addiction Research in the Classic Era of Narcotic Control* (Baltimore: The Johns Hopkins University Press, 2002).

[22] M. Houlbrook, *Queer London: Perils and Pleasures in the Sexual Metropolis, 1918–1957* (London: University of Chicago Press, 2005). Matt Houlbrook's is an account of queer sexuality and does not deal with drugs. It should be noted, moreover, that Houlbrook rejects the use of the term 'subculture' in his work. He states: 'In the lives they forged in London's public, commercial, and residential spaces and in the ways in which they made sense of their desires and practices, men were never a distinct subculture somehow removed from the city, but an integral part of modern metropolitan life.' p. 264. I would argue that most subcultures were not 'somehow removed from the city' but deeply integrated in it, as Chaps. 3 and 4 will show. Regardless of this, I shall use the terms interchangeably.

been seen as bereft of subculture, with the respectable therapeutic addict on one side and the artistic cliques with their drug-based gestures on the other. The research has identified an opiate subculture that posseses much in common with that of the 1960s addicts, albeit with some important differences, especially centred on the role of women. It finds prototypical script doctors, the forerunners of those who were believed to be a postwar phenomenon, already practising their marginal medicine during the First World War, and introduces the strands of a cultural narrative surrounding drug that subsequent chapters trace across the lifetime of the classical 'British System'.

Outline of the Book

Chapter 2 maps the emergence and cultural geography of the script doctor, making use of two case studies. One shorter study examines the practice of a Bond Street physician prescribing heroin to the wife of an officer in the Royal Flying Corps, and provides an account of ways in which the growing problem of drug prescribing constituted a lacuna in the control system enshrined in DORA 40b, and subsequently the Dangerous Drugs Acts of 1920s and 1923, which clamped down with considerable success on the proto-subcultures of cocaine and opium consumption in the early 1920s. The second case study is a longer one, tracing the career of Dr Samuel Connor, a major script doctor figure whose prescribing haunted (and played a large part in prompting) the Rolleston Committee, the deliberations of which resulted in the report that laid the foundations of the regulatory regime for the next 50 years—the classic 'British System'. Connor's marginal practice brought together sexual and narcotic medicine, as well as the subcultures of these closely related issues. The problem of identifying nontherapeutic addicts, devising appropriate forms of treatment and regulating doctors' dealings with this difficult population was central to the Rolleston Committee and was a recurring theme in the regulatory discourse through the classic period of addiction treatment.

Chapter 3 examines the appearance and characteristics of an opiate subculture in the early 1930s. Basing the analysis on the case of Brenda Dean Paul, it traces the consolidation of this white drug culture from upper-class bohemia. The erosion of the aristocracy's social and political power created new cultural spaces for elite youth, who enjoyed transnational links with other metropolitan centres and their bohemias and modernisms: London, Paris, Berlin, New York. Several of those at the centre of the 'bright young people' crossed over into an emerging drug subculture, embracing pleasure and sexual experimentation and rejecting an Englishness that represented to them the repression of these categories. The chapter explores this new set, its subcultural spaces, its relations to doctors and treatments and its court cases. It also analyses its drug subcultural discourse by reference to memoirs and so on and especially to an anonymous postcard sent to Mr Griffith Jones, a magistrate who in 1932 sent BDP to prison. The postcard defends drug use in feminist and ecological terms.

Chapter 4 explores a second, rather different heroin, subculture of the later 1930s. Emerging not from bohemia but rather from the 'West End life', that subculture of London's pleasure and entertainment district, this subculture was closer to the underworld of the night-time economy, drawn from a mixed class background (upper, middle and working classes), entrepreneurial and predominantly heterosexual. It was based in the nightclubs and bottle parties of Mayfair and Soho. Heroin was the preferred opiate and was usually sniffed (rather than injected) at social events known in the press as heroin snuff parties. This group derived its drugs illicitly from Paris and used cannabis and cocaine in addition to heroin. Its leading figure was Gerry O'Brien, an uncle of Garret FitzGerald, later the Irish Premier. The chapter compares and contrasts the two 1930s opiate subcultures and their relationships with the control networks; it considers the complexity of drug subcultures and their relationships with sexual and criminal metropolitan subcultures.

Chapter 5 traces the early history of the Home Office Drugs Branch and the network of regulatory agencies that cooperated to try to curtail the activities of those groups and individuals using opiates for 'nontherapeutic' purposes. These included the Metropolitan Police (the focus is mainly on London because the subculture was increasingly performed there), the Chemist Inspection Officers and the specialist Drugs Officers who were the predecessors of the Drugs Squad formed after the Second World War, and finally the Regional Medical Officers who cooperated with the Home Office Drugs Branch to investigate cases of heavy or extended prescribing identified by the Chemist Inspection Offices. (NB: The Pharmaceutical Society was also involved in regulating chemist shops but was not greatly involved with script doctors or consumers.) A complex and dense network of forces sought to regulate both drug consumers and the doctors whose prescribing formed their major source of supply, though—as we will see in the next chapter—there were channels of illicit supply that brought opiates to consumers in London, especially from Paris. The regulatory agencies worked cooperatively, though there were often tensions between them over specific issues. Other forces also contributed to the suppression of drug use: various members of the public such as cab drivers, messenger boys, servants, hotel managers and so on. I call this the 'lay culture of surveillance'.

Chapter 6 examines the growing dissatisfaction amongst doctors and addiction experts in medicine, psychiatry, the prisons and government departments (Home Office, Ministry of Health). These discontents led to the setting up of the Royal College of Physicians Committee on Drug Addiction in 1938 and are reflected in its workings. The composition of the Committee was strongly influenced by eugenics, and its establishment was initiated by eugenicists in the medical and allied professions. Discussions were mainly structured around the perceived need to confine and segregate the addict population; the core issue was whether to stop at addicts or to lock up the entire population of misfits—the deviant nation. This was an old theme in addiction discourse. The Home Office was ambivalent about the proposals but finally came down against them. The anti-segregation wing of the Committee was led by Russell Brain, who went on to chair two influential committees on addiction in the twilight years of the classic British System. In many ways the last push of the British eugenics movement, the RCP Committee, did not produce a final report, being stymied by internal conflicts and the outbreak of war. However, the theme of addict confinement resurfaced at the Home Office following the Second World War when new criminal justice legislation was thought to offer a means of incarcerating addicts who had committed no criminal offence.

In Chap. 7, the threat of air raids in the build-up to the Second World War is explored. This led many in medicine and politics to anticipate 'mass hysteria' amongst the population on the Home Front. This left the Home Office Drugs Branch facing a new and somewhat unprecedented challenge: how to regulate morphine when the drug was widely and densely distributed across the social body and many doctors advocated using the drug in a therapeutic capacity to guard against civilian panic. This alarmed a Drugs Branch staff accustomed to restricting access to opiates, and led to tensions with the Ministry of Health, which supported a broad relaxation of controls. Meanwhile, the new wartime proliferation of licit opiates offered opportunities to the addict population, who were quick to infiltrate the civil defence system with a view to accessing supplies. Another key wartime development was the advent of Dr Quinlan, a major script doctor who proved able to remain continually beyond the reach of the regulatory authorities, and offers an example of the consolidation of the script doctor in inner London. In this period, changes in the addict subculture begin to be apparent.

Chapter 8 re-examines the 'postwar boom' in opiate addiction, in which sociological research has identified the first appearance of drug subculture in Britain. The changes that characterised the postwar years are reassessed, and it is argued that the rapid increase in heroin users was not a matter of an opiate subculture appearing in place of the pre-war medicalised addicts, nor of script doctors taking over from normative practitioners. Rather, one wave of London's opiate subculture morphed into another, larger grouping, which was linked with the youth culture arriving as part of the more developed consumer society of the 1950s. This new subculture took over the characteristic spaces of the earlier subculture of the 1930s, the nightclubs, cafes and bars of Soho, and drew on the practical drug know-how of the previous subcultural addicts. In addition, the building up of an established body of script doctors over some 25 years provided the drug availability necessary to equip the postwar proliferation of addiction, underpinning the market until the latter part of the 1960s. This period also saw the radical changes in the organisation of the Met's chemist inspection work, a development the Drugs Branch had been seeking since the 1920s. These changes meant that much more reliable data could be fed into the Addicts Index, which was overwhelmingly based on the work of the Chemist Inspection Officers.

Chapter 9 represents the conclusion of the text, brings together and updates the themes explored throughout the previous chapters and revises the picture of opiate subculture and its relationships to the British System, which have been based chiefly on sociological work. The opiate drug culture of the 1960s is seen as a development of earlier groups, trends and attitudes taking place across the lifespan of the classic British System. It inhabited the same iconic spaces as its 1930s predecessor, and had recourse to a tradition of script doctors that had been evolving in parallel with British opiate consumption since before the Rolleston Report. This second wave of opiate subculture expanded and proliferated in ways that the first wave was unable to, because the social and cultural context had changed, and was much less restrictive. The spread of broadly bohemian attitudes and practices through the host society brought the opiate subculture and its values closer to those of the cultural mainstream, while the British System of prescribing was largely, if gradually, consigned to the past by the changes stemming from the second Brain Committee.

CHAPTER 2

From Injudicious Prescribing to the Script Doctor: Transgressive Addiction Treatment in the Interwar Years

Introduction

This chapter traces the emergence, evolution and consolidation of the figure of the 'script doctor'. This was a term that originated within the institutional discourse of the Home Office Drugs Branch in the 1930s. It referred to a practitioner whom the Home Office believed supplied drugs to addicts merely to pander to the passion for drugs: not in the course of bona fide medical treatment aimed at achieving an abstinence-based cure but 'simply to satisfy their craving'—a prescription in exchange for a fee.[1] Doses were high, and the spirit and often the detail of the regulations were disregarded in multiple ways; the motivation of the physician was assumed to be pecuniary. A further key characteristic of the script doctor was the perceived tendency to cultivate an addict clientele made up of those belonging to the 'underworld'—or what Sir William Willcox, medical advisor to the Home Office in the 1920s and 1930s, called the 'vicious group' of addicts.[2,3]

[1] Departmental Committee on Morphine and Heroin Addiction, *Report* (London: HMSO, 1926) Para.10.

[2] W. J. Bishop, 'Willcox, Sir William Henry (1870–1941)', rev. K. D. Watson, *Oxford Dictionary of National Biography*, (Oxford: Oxford University Press, 2004). [http://www.oxforddnb.com/view/article/36910, accessed 11 Nov 2015].

[3] W. H. Willcox, 'Norman Kerr Memorial Lecture On Drug Addiction. Delivered Before The Society For The Study Of Inebriety, October 9th, 1923' *British Medical Journal* 2, 3283 (1923) pp. 1013–1018.

C. Hallam, *White Drug Cultures and Regulation in London, 1916–1960*, https://doi.org/10.1007/978-3-319-94770-9_2

Some researchers have contended that the advent of these doctors coincided with the arrival of the 'junkie' subculture in the 1950s. According to Judith Blackwell, 'the new heroin users had imported an essentially American role model and…"conning a quack" was a skill that was part of the performance of that role'. She went on to say that, '"Script doctors" are an integral part of the lore of American junkies.'[4] In fact, the nomenclature is foreign to the US heroin culture and had its institutional birth in the UK. While it has proved impossible to identify any precise date of origin, the term was in use at the Home Office during the 1930s, and from there was picked up by the Metropolitan Police; it was, for example, mentioned in a lecture delivered to the police by Home Office Drugs Branch Inspector Selby-Boothroyd in 1938 and featured in several of the Branch's subsequent annual reports.[5,6,7]

The historiographic starting point for this research, and for any research in the field and period, is the posthumously published work of H. B. 'Bing' Spear, who worked at the Home Office Drugs Branch for over 30 years.[8] Spear provided a narrative of the conduct of injudicious prescribers from the 1920s on, though he remarked, no doubt accurately, that 'it is not now possible to be certain about the chronology'.[9] Certainly, there were practising script doctors whom Spear failed to mention. The Home Office practice of destroying old files relating to doctors is probably to blame for

[4] J. Blackwell, 'The Saboteurs of Britain's Opiate Policy: Overprescribing Physicians or American-Style 'Junkies'?' *The International Journal of the Addictions,* 23,5 (1988) pp. 517–526.

[5] To date, the earliest identified reference to the term appears in a London lecture given in 1933 to the Society for the Study of Addiction by Dr Pablo Wolff. Wolff refers to 'so-called script doctors', and I believe it is likely that he is using the Home Office's own term; several eminent medical figures associated with the Home Office, including Willcox, were in attendance. But there is at present no external evidence to support this reading. See P. Wolff, 'Alcohol and Drug Addiction in Germany: Part 2- Drug Addiction' *British Journal of Inebriety* 30, 4 (1933) pp. 160–171.

[6] HO 45/18469, 'The Work of the Drugs Branch'. Notes for lecture given by C. B. Selby-Boothroyd, Home Office D. D. Inspector, at the 8th District Detective Conference, 29 June 1938.

[7] HO 45/24948 'Annual Report of Home Office Drugs Branch for 1940'.

[8] H. B. Spear, *Heroin Addiction, Care and Control.* Another work by Spear that covers substantially the same ground is 'The early years of Britain's drug situation in practice: up to the 1960s' in J. Strang & M. Gossop, (eds), *Heroin Addiction and the British System: Volume 1: Origins and Evolution* (London & New York, Routledge, 2002).

[9] H. B. Spear, *Heroin Addiction, Care and Control.* p. 51.

the patchy state of surviving records.[10] Spear's account is essentially no more than a short sketch, though it does provide an invaluable set of references, forming a point of departure for further research into this neglected domain. Less usefully, Spear takes the Home Office version of these prescribers as read, viewing them unproblematically as mere traders in prescriptions. He goes some way toward linking them with some of their better-known drug-consuming patients, though again the connections are sketchy. Given the shortage of materials, this is perhaps inevitable. However, there are in Spear's work a number of factual errors concerning the interwar drug consumers; while these are relatively minor, they cast doubt on some of the more important linkages made by Spear. In particular, he states that Dr Arthur Edwin Tait prescribed drugs for several of the O'Brien group in the late 1930s. I have found nothing in support of this claim, though Tait was undoubtedly a significant 'script doctor'.[11]

In addition to Home Office documents, this chapter makes use of journalistic sources to draw out the social and cultural context of the doctors and their addict clients. In addition, the Metropolitan Police files concerning Brenda Dean Paul provide a rich source of information that was apparently unavailable to Spear and which helps us to understand the relationships obtaining between practitioners and patients, albeit viewed through the lens of police discourse and practices.

The 1930s: A Key Decade

In addition to its historiographic status as the inception of the quiet times, the 1930s was a key decade in the wider development of Britain's drug scene, and a period of consolidation in a number of important ways. The Drugs Branch itself, which had hitherto consisted of an ad hoc arrangement at the Home Office, became in 1933 a more or less permanent institutional edifice with a defined brief. At about the same time, an opiate subculture emerged from the drug-consuming elements of high bohemia in Chelsea and within the night-time economy of the West End, and included groupings that endured over subsequent decades and conveyed a body of practical drug knowledge to the new wave of heroin users that appeared in the 1950s. Lastly, as noted above, the 1930s saw the 'formal'

[10] TNA HO 319/14, 'Survey of the results of Home Office policy in combating addiction during the period 1st January 1946 to 31st December 1953', p. 1.

[11] Dr Tait is discussed on p. 70.

arrival upon the scene of the script doctor, a personage intimately interwoven with both the Home Office and the white drug culture, each of which depended upon the others and, as it were, kept them in business.[12] However, the pattern of practice that characterised these script doctors had largely developed before the 1930s and predated the nomenclature; the opportunistic supplying of drugs by doctors was underway as early as 1917 to white drug consumers who appear to have rejected the medical model and evolved over the ensuing decade. The chain of supply crystallised in the 1930s and was by then unambiguously centred on London, drawing consumers from around the country to the increasingly cosmopolitan capital. This development was in part a result of the proximity of the opiate and cocaine culture that was forming there, and in part derived from the social and economic changes affecting the Harley Street medical district, changes whose influence seems to have been felt in medicine across the West End and inner London. From this point on, the classic era of the British System was characterised by the continuing presence of script doctors, who constituted the primary source of drug supply for the drug culture that they helped to create. The present chapter focuses on some of those cases that constituted milestones in the development of 'injudicious prescribing' and the attempts of the regulatory authorities to deal with it.[13]

The Regulatory Background

Around the industrialised world, restrictive drug laws had been introduced, and the problems that the authorities associated with what would later be called the 'maintenance' supply of drugs to addicts were being considered and addressed. The example of the USA was one of several that had been monitored closely by the Home Office. In the US, the prescribing of maintenance supplies had been effectively outlawed by a Supreme Court decision taken in 1919. As one physician with legal expertise remarked, 'The result has been that no matter how acute the sufferings of an addict might be, incident to the partial or total withdrawal of his or her drug, the average physician was afraid to do anything to bring about relief,

[12] 'White drugs' was a contemporary term for powdered drugs such as heroin, morphine and cocaine, as opposed to opium and cannabis. There is further discussion of this term at the beginning of Chap. 3.

[13] TNA HO144/11913, 'Home Office to R. H. Crooke, Secretary to the Departmental Committee 14 November 1924' and 'Home Office Memorandum', 'Cases included as "Injudicious" Prescribing etc.' Undated.

lest he be summoned into court and held up to public obloquy as a "dope pedlar".'[14] Despite a modification of the Supreme Court's position on the maintenance question in the Linder case of 1925, these fears were now embedded in the American medical profession and shaped its treatment of addiction. Consequently, US addicts turned exclusively to the rapidly expanding illicit market in order to obtain supplies.[15]

The situation in Britain, meanwhile, remained in flux; under both DORA and the 1920 Dangerous Drugs Act, the interpretation of the law in relation to the supply of drugs to addicts by doctors was unsettled, and a range of treatment practices characterised the responses of UK physicians.[16] Most of those in general practice, it must be recalled, might pass their careers without ever encountering such florid modern pathologies as opiate addiction; those that did were mostly located in metropolitan districts. Though addicts were widely distributed geographically, it was those who consumed drugs for entertainment and pleasure who clustered together in the large cities, and it was the doctors servicing this deviant population that were considered problematic by the Home Office.

Any duly qualified doctor could prescribe drugs such as morphine, heroin and cocaine for a patient, including for the treatment of addiction.[17] The Dangerous Drugs Act confirmed the authority of a medical practitioner to possess and supply dangerous drugs 'so far as is necessary for the practice of his profession'.[18] There was, however, no further definition contained in the regulations, and no obvious way in which the authorities might distinguish 'bona fide' medical practice from its transgressive counterpart; though addiction had been successfully claimed by medicine, its therapies remained uncertain, and no consensus drew out the contours of an authoritatively approved clinical response.

[14] W. C. Woodward, 'The Supreme Court Decision in Linder vs. United States- as it affects the Harrison Narcotic Act' Californian *and Western Medicine* 24,3 (1926) pp. 362–364.

[15] D. Courtwright 'The Roads to H: The Emergence of the American Heroin Complex, 1898–1956' in D. F. Musto (ed.) *One Hundred Years of Heroin* (London: Auburn House, 2002).

[16] Malcolm, M.T. 'Morphine Withdrawal, Treatments 1900–1930' History *of Psychiatry,*10,37 (1999) pp. 13–26.

[17] At this point, it was not unusual for doctors to dispense drugs to patients. When the term 'prescribing' is used as it is in this sentence, it should be understood in the broader sense of 'supply', which could include prescribing proper (i.e. giving a prescription that could be dispensed by a pharmacist) and dispensing (handing the drugs over to a patient directly or administering an injection). Where a more precise meaning is required, this will be indicated.

[18] The Regulations under the Dangerous Drugs Act of 1920. Regulation 5.

As shown by Berridge, during the period immediately following the passage of the 1920 Act, the Home Office itself conceptualised the 'cure' of addiction as involving either the abrupt cessation of supplies or a more gradual reduction of dosage leading to zero.[19] Consequently, the supply of what are currently known as 'maintenance' doses did not correspond to the Home Office model of what constituted proper medical treatment. And the problem confronted the Home Office with increasing urgency: what could be done about injudicious prescribing?

Injudicious Prescribing

The category of injudicious prescribing as conceptualised by the Home Office was a broad one, and various kinds of cases tended to come under its heading. In the main, they can be resolved into three subtypes, to which I shall refer as the *compassionate*, the *eccentric* and the *transgressive*. Clearly, there is blurring and overlap between such analytical typologies, but they do nonetheless correspond with the main ways in which the complex realities of actual cases were viewed and handled by the authorities in the immediate pre-Rolleston era.[20] The two former types, the compassionate and the eccentric, would typically involve only one or two cases of addiction amongst a doctor's clientele. Such examples generally involved professional individuals who complied with contemporary medical understandings of addiction, were scattered across the country and were usually isolated from other addicts. I will briefly consider the compassionate and eccentric prescriber before moving on to the transgressive modality.

The compassionate prescriber is exemplified in the well-known case of the painter and photographic tutor Thomas Henderson, whose addiction predated the Dangerous Drugs Acts and enabled him to carry on his profession and lead a 'useful life'.[21] At the time of his dealings with the Home

[19] V. Berridge, "Stamping out addiction': the work of the Rolleston Committee 1924–1926' in G. E. Berrios, & H. Freeman (eds), *150 Years of British Psychiatry Volume 2: The Aftermath* (London: Athlone, 1996).

[20] The Rolleston Committee, which reported in 1926, set the parameters for addiction treatment and elaborated the basis of the 'British System'. See Chap. 1.

[21] TNA HO 144/11913, 'Thomas Henderson to Home Office, 20 November 1922'. For historians' discussions of the case, see V. Berridge, *Opium and the People: Opiate Use and Drug Control Policy in Nineteenth and Early Twentieth Century England* (London: Free Association Books, 1999) pp. 270–272. See also H. Padwa, *Social Poison: The Culture and Politics of Opiate Control in Britain and France, 1891–1926*. (Baltimore: Johns Hopkins University Press, 2012) pp. 154–157.

Office, Henderson was being treated by Dr J. S. Robertson, whom Permanent Undersecretary of State Sir Malcolm Delevingne, who was in charge of drugs issues at the Home Office, described as a 'very mediocre practitioner in a poor quarter at the other side of London'.[22] Dr Robertson practised at Walworth Road in South London, which was in fact a short geographical distance from the Home Office at Queen Anne's Chambers—though these two locations were culturally remote from one another. Despite Delevingne's scathing opinion of Robertson, the Home Office inquiry into the Henderson case did not result in an intervention, though it was a close-run thing. It no doubt helped that when Sir William Willcox interviewed the patient in the company of Dr Robertson, his report spoke of the latter in appreciative terms, and found nothing to suggest that the practitioner was motivated by anything other than a genuine concern for his difficult patient.[23]

A less well-known instance of what I am calling compassionate prescribing is that of Dr J. B. Mainprize of Sheffield, who wrote to the Home Office in December 1922 to ask the advice of officials regarding an unnamed patient who had been a laudanum drinker since long before the 1920 Act. 'When her supply was stopped by the chemist she collapsed and called me in', Mainprize explained. He had tried a range of substitutes for Mrs X, as he labelled her, but was eventually forced to revert to a supply of opium, which he considered essential for maintaining the patient's health. 'Am I doing wrong?' he pleaded. 'I cannot get a satisfactory answer from my solicitor.'[24] Here too the prescriber appeared to be motivated entirely by the healthcare needs of the patient, and reluctantly supplied the drug in order to forestall a collapse. In such cases, which were relatively common, the Home Office generally appears to have taken no further action beyond monitoring the ongoing situation. Mrs X was probably the only addict on Dr Mainprize's books; he had been candid regarding the details of the case and the legal grey area into which he was concerned it might lead him. The case did, nonetheless, form a part of that range of ambivalent relationships between doctor and addict patient that led the Home Office to seek the support of the medical profession, and eventually

[22] TNA MH 71/108, 'Home Office Memorandum to the Departmental Committee, Appendix 1. Case number 18'.

[23] TNA MH 71/108, 'Home Office Memorandum to the Departmental Committee, Appendix 1. Case number 18'. The papers include a report of the examination by Sir William Willcox.

[24] TNA HO 45/11285, 'Dr Mainprize to Home Office.' 5 December 1922.

the Ministry of Health and the Rolleston Committee, in its attempt to establish a clear dividing line between what it understood as bona fide medical treatment on the one hand and, on the other, the enabling of a degenerate habit.

The eccentric prescriber, meanwhile, is ably represented by the example of Dr Grant, a Glasgow practitioner known locally as the 'daft doctor'.[25] As a result of a chemist shop inspection by the Glasgow police which revealed his prescribing of large quantities of morphine and cocaine to one George Ellis, Dr Grant was visited by Dr Cullen of the Scottish Board of Health; Cullen was the equivalent of the English Regional Medical Officer (RMO).[26] Ellis was an amputee, having lost a leg at the age of 15, and suffered recurrent pain as a consequence. He was a masseur by profession, also offering electrical stimulation as a therapeutic treatment. Dr Grant had been supplying Ellis with prescriptions for drugs for around two years, and, though they permitted him to carry on his working life, Dr Cullen was convinced that these supplies were issued primarily to support his addiction. Dr Grant had a previous history of supplying large quantities and strange combinations of drugs and had been surcharged repeatedly under the National Health Insurance scheme for his prescribing excesses.[27] There is no mention of any further addicts amongst his clientele, and his local reputation for odd behaviour is supported by the description Dr Cullen drew of his chaotic surgery and practice.

Practitioners in this grouping were sometimes of advanced age and had frequently qualified several decades previously; consequently, they were

[25] TNA HO 45/11285, 'Report in regard to Dr Donald John Collan Grant, 168 Stirling Road, Glasgow', 6 January 1923. It is noteworthy that this 'daft doctor' sobriquet has caused some historiographic confusion, for when the case papers were condensed for inclusion in the Home Office documents provided for the consideration of the Rolleston Committee, it was wrongly transcribed as 'draft doctor', a slip of the bureaucratic pen that subsequently led historian Howard Padwa to conclude that such practitioners were known generically as 'draft doctors'. Transcribing errors apart, there is no evidence that this was the case, and these practitioners remained without a specific moniker until the advent of the term 'script doctors' in the subsequent decade. See H. Padwa, *Social Poison: The Culture and Politics of Opiate Control in Britain and France, 1891–1926* (Baltimore: Johns Hopkins University Press, 2012) p. 154.

[26] Regional medical officers had been given the authority to inspect doctor's records in 1922 and worked to support the Home Office in cases that suggested injudicious prescribing. For further details, see Chap. 4.

[27] TNA HO 45/11285, 'Report in regard to Dr Donald John Collan Grant, 168 Stirling Road, Glasgow', 6 January 1923.

often unaware of recent therapeutic developments. The Home Office appears to have varied in its responses to eccentric prescribing, though insufficient records have survived to provide a detailed picture. Grant's record-keeping failures were so flagrant that it offered the Home Office the opportunity to prosecute, which if successful would have given it the right to withdraw his authority to possess and supply dangerous drugs. Grant—perhaps not so 'daft' in this respect at least—had quickly brought his records up to date, which effectively removed the opportunity to prosecute. Dr Cullen's report, however, suggests that other grounds might have been identified, and it is probable that Grant was a borderline case in terms of the level of Home Office concern it provoked. Such decisions were made on a case-by-case basis and reflected the absence of clear grounds on which to decide them.

The final grouping of injudicious prescribers, and the one of greatest interest for this research, is that of the transgressive prescriber. These were the practitioners who marked out the pattern of supply that caused most concern to the Home Office, right from these formative years to the close of the classic period of the British System in the mid-1960s. They were doctors who, according to the Home Office, prescribed drugs with no real reference to a therapeutic project, who flouted the regulations by demanding only occasional face-to-face consultations with clients and by regularly posting prescriptions and supplies of drugs; they would increase dosage on request and keep inadequate records or none. Moreover, they were suspected of being attracted to addict patients primarily by the prospect of large and regular fees. This pattern of practice evolved along with the regulatory architecture through the 1920s and 1930s but was present from the earliest days of legal regulation under the Defence of the Realm Act regulation 40b.

Dr Reginald Nitch Smith: Transgressive Practice Under DORA 40b

The first case of a doctor caught up in the legal ramifications that surrounded the prescribing and dispensing framework occurred in 1917, and involved Dr Reginald Nitch Smith of New Bond Street W1, a surgeon and physician who had practised in the West End since 1899. The case came under the auspices of DORA 40b. It followed on from an earlier court appearance by Mrs Deborah Platt, a heroin addict and the wife of an officer in the Coldstream Guards.

Deborah Platt, accompanied by an attending nurse, appeared at Marlborough Street police court in July 1917 charged with seven cases of jewellery theft involving items stolen from jewellers in New Bond Street and around the West End. Mrs Platt's court appearance was unusual for her high-class position; she was the daughter of an elite military family, living with her husband at Buckingham Gate in Belgravia, where they were attended by 11 servants including 2 footmen.[28,29] Deborah Platt's lady's maid had uncovered her mistress' addiction by finding a hidden syringe and some tubes of heroin tablets, and testified in some detail to all of this in court.[30] She was quoted as explaining that 'when her mistress took the drug she used to lock herself in a room', adding that the first effect of the drug was excitement, followed by a depression that drove back to her syringe.[31] It is difficult not to detect a whiff of class vengeance in the witness' testimony, and this lurid scene of upper-class decadence was to become more familiar in the drug cases of the early 1930s.

It is unclear whether the jewellery thefts were connected with the funding of her heroin use or were undertaken for pleasure or rebellion in their own right, but either way, when the case was transferred to the Old Bailey, in addition to binding her over, the judge directed that the physician from whom she had obtained the drugs should be brought before the General Medical Council (GMC) on charges of professional misconduct. The overall impression that emerged from the courtroom was that Mrs Platt was the victim, while the Bond Street doctor was the villain of the piece.

When the case of 'infamous conduct in a professional respect' came before the GMC in December 1917, there were two charges. First, that Dr Nitch Smith had sold drugs at exorbitant prices and other than in the course of medical treatment and that, knowing that Deborah Platt was addicted, he continued supplying her to her moral and physical detriment.

[28] Ross McKibbin has drawn attention to the conflicted relations between domestic servants and their employers at the end of the First World War; these were on view in the courtroom. It was Catherine Bradley, Mrs Platt's lady's maid, who informed police of her mistress's habit of heroin injecting and directed them to the stolen jewellery. For the general trend of conflict between upper classes and their servants, see R. McKibbin, *Classes and Cultures: England 1918–1951* (Oxford: Oxford University Press, 2000) p. 61.

[29] W. Bridge, *Captain Henry Evelyn Arthur Platt—Diaries and Letters of a First World War Officer* (CreateSpace Independent Publishing Platform, Amazon.com, 2012) pp. 101–103.

[30] *Birmingham Daily Post* 16 July 1917, p. 7. See also *Times* 30 November 1917, p. 10; *Daily Express* 29 November 1917, p. 8 & *Daily Express* 30 November 1917, p. 8.

[31] *Birmingham Daily Post* 16 July 1917, p. 7.

Second, by supplying the drugs, which were allegedly destined for an officer and men of the British Armed Forces, he had contravened regulation 40 of the Defence of the Realm Act and the Army Council order of May 11, 1916, which prohibited the sale or gift of intoxicants to military personnel. It should be recalled that at this juncture heroin itself was not controlled under DORA 40b, and consequently Mrs Platt did not face specific charges in relation to her possession of the drug. The source of the problem was seen as lying with the physician, who had supplied her with large quantities of heroin and charged her the sum of £137 over a period of several months.[32] In providing Deborah Platt with heroin, a taste for which she had, like so many others, first picked up in France, the doctor had contravened the guidelines governing the medical profession. At the GMC hearing, Deborah Platt retracted her statement that some of the heroin was bound for her husband's military unit in France, a move that effectively left the doctor facing only the professional charges against him.

Nitch Smith told the Council that he had 'many drug-takers under his care'.[33] His counsel noted that Deborah Platt had obtained additional heroin by deceiving several other doctors and argued that Nitch Smith was being used as a 'whipping post' in relation to her jewellery thefts.[34] Nonetheless, the doctor was found guilty of infamous conduct in a professional respect and his name erased from the medical register.

Transgressive Prescribing: The GMC and the Problem Facing the Home Office

To summarise the argument thus far: at the heart of the Home Office's difficulties lay the problem of curtailing what it regarded as the transgressive prescriber. Under both DORA 40b and the subsequent Dangerous Drugs Acts, the Home Secretary had the power to withdraw a doctor's authority to possess and supply dangerous drugs *once he or she had been convicted of an offence under the Act.* This became the Home Office's preferred method of dealing with the transgressive prescriber; it was rapid and involved little interagency or bureaucratic cooperation. However, it was of no use in those cases where a practitioner was sufficiently careful to fulfil

[32] 'Supply of Drugs by Doctor to Patient who had formed the Drug Habit'. *British Medical Journal* (Supplement) 2,2971 (1917) p. 114.

[33] Ibid.

[34] *Birmingham Daily Post* 30 November 1917, p. 7.

the demands of the regulations. The dangerous drugs legislation included no limits to dosage and indeed left the treatment entirely up to the doctor's professional and clinical judgement so long as he or she complied with the record-keeping and prescription requirements.

The Nitch Smith case is significant as an early example of the transgressive prescriber, or what the Home Office Drugs Branch would, in the 1930s, term the script doctor. It is also notable in that it represents the only case during the classic period of the British System in which the GMC provided the direct mechanism, through its disciplinary committee, for stopping the activities of the transgressive prescriber by striking his name from the medical register. The subsequent involvement of the Council was, prior to the 1970s, restricted to cases in which practitioners had already been convicted of dangerous drugs offences and had their authority removed by the Home Secretary.[35]

As noted above, the Home Office was confronted with a number of cases of injudicious prescribing in the immediate pre-Rolleston years.[36] Reginald Nitch Smith's relatively short-lived foray into transgressive prescribing gave some indication of the problematic potential of the system, but the arrival on the scene of Dr Samuel Grahame Connor represented a quantum leap in the evolution of deviant medical practice, specialising in an underworld addict clientele and operating on a scale that Nitch Smith never approached.

The Case of Dr Connor: 'A London Doctor Who Is Notorious for Giving Drug Prescriptions'[37]

Samuel Grahame Connor was born in Newry, Northern Ireland, on August 24, 1865, into a large middle-class family, his father being the justice of the peace in that town. He qualified in Edinburgh in 1889 (M.B.C.M.) and began practising in the West End of London in 1893. He came first to the attention of the Home Office in 1919 when he was providing supplies of cocaine to a known addict, thereby beginning a long

[35] S. G. Mars, *The Politics of Addiction: Medical Conflict and Drug Dependence in England since the 1960s* (Basingstoke: Palgrave Macmillan, 2012) p. 66.

[36] The Home Office informed R. H. Crooke, secretary to the Rolleston Committee, that it had details of 45 cases of injudicious prescribing. See TNA HO 144/11913, 'Home Office to Crooke, 14 November 1924'.

[37] TNA MH 58/277, Appendix 1. Case 25.

career as a thorn in the side of the regulatory system.[38] In time he came to haunt the Home Office's drugs staff, and the proceedings of the Departmental Committee on Morphine and Heroin Addiction when it began its deliberations in 1924.

The Home Office had noted, through its inspections of large pharmaceutical distributors, that Connor was purchasing sizeable amounts of cocaine for practice use; the substance, he claimed, was employed as an anaesthetic in the treatment of venereal disease. Records of the police involvement of 1919 provide a first signal that Connor's practice included addicts and those requiring services related to sex—those two areas of medical practice that would bring him into almost continuous conflict with the regulatory authorities until his death in February 1941.

These services were important to many of the patients that surrounded Dr Connor in his professional life, the social and cultural geography of which is significant. His practice was located on the edge of Soho at Dryden Chambers, a four-storey block and courtyard reached by means of an archway on the south side of Oxford Street, adjacent to yet hidden from the crowds of shoppers. As Marek Kohn has shown, the West End and Soho area represented the cradle of new forms of drug consumption and the networks and styles of sociability that went with them.[39] A search of contemporary records shows the mix of people living at Dryden Chambers when Connor was practising there. His neighbours were amongst those who served the theatres and cinemas, clubs and hotels as dressmakers, musicians, composers, theatrical agents, advertisers and all the associated trades of the West End pleasure district.[40] They also included the 'wide' community that made its living by exploiting the district.[41] By locating his consulting rooms here, Dr Connor had found the perfect location to practise a medicine of the margins. Those who were engaging in hedonistic lifestyles and required a physician who would offer a menu of services that responded to their drug use and addictions, their

[38] TNA MH 58/277, Appendix 1. Case 1, and MEPO 3/1023, 'REX V. Samuel Grahame Connor: Particulars of cases coming to the notice of Police, taken from CID correspondence'.

[39] M. Kohn, *Dope Girls, passim.*

[40] The type of businesses based around Dryden Court can be viewed in the notices of *The London Gazette.* For a discussion of the Soho district, see J. R. Walkowitz, *Nights Out: Life in Cosmopolitan London* (New Haven & London: Yale University Press, 2012).

[41] M. Benney, *Low Company: Describing the evolution of a burglar* (London: Caliban, 1981; first published in 1936).

transgressive sexual behaviours, with associated venereal infections and requirements for contraception and abortion, could easily and discreetly access Connor's practice.

Over the ensuing years, Connor acquired a dubious reputation. A West End pharmacist had informed the police that Connor was seeing 'men and women of the underworld' and had 'three or four hundred addict patients of this class'.[42] He was visited by the police on behalf of the Home Office and 'asked to be more careful in regard to the prescriptions he gave for Dangerous Drugs…'.[43] On this occasion, the Met's solicitors 'did not consider prosecution advisable', despite the fact that officers had identified prescriptions that contained technical irregularities. It was a decision that the Home Office would later regret, as a conviction would have offered them their preferred option of deploying the Dangerous Drugs Acts in order to withdraw Connor's authority to possess and supply drugs.

Further misdemeanours quickly followed: Connor was implicated in abortions, and Brighton Police surgeon Dr Pulling reported that a local addict had overdosed on cocaine that he had obtained on the doctor's prescription.[44] Shortly afterwards, Connor received a formal visit from a Regional Medical Officer. In the words of the Home Office, he 'admitted prescribing Cocaine to addicts purely for the satisfaction of their addiction. He expressed his thanks when the R.M.O. advised him that this was an improper proceeding, and gave a written undertaking to prescribe, in future only for "such cases as I can treat"'.[45] The use of a written undertaking, though it had no force in law, was a tactic that the Home Office employed frequently in its dealings with transgressive prescribers and doctor addicts as an alternative to prosecution.[46] Often, however, it turned out to be merely another step in an escalating response from the authorities, and such was the case with Connor.

Shortly afterwards, another prosecution involving some of his addict patients took place at Marlborough Street. The case received considerable publicity, partly because the accused were suffering so badly from withdrawal symptoms following a night in the police cells that they were unable

[42] TNA MH 58/277, Appendix 1. Case 1.

[43] *Times* 17 April 1926, p. 9.

[44] TNA MEPO 3/1023, 'REX V. Samuel Grahame Connor: Particulars of cases coming to the notice of Police, taken from CID correspondence'.

[45] TNA MH 58/277, Appendix 1. Case 1.

[46] H. B. Spear, *Heroin Addiction, Care and Control*, p. 49.

to stand up and had to be carried from the courtroom.[47] The prosecuting counsel judged that the defendants, who were of independent means, were 'saturated with drugs' and 'in a hopeless state of moral and physical decay'.[48] In early 1924 Connor was, on the advice of the Director of Public Prosecutions, given a formal warning as to his conduct in the treatment of addicts.[49]

Despite this litany of infractions, Connor continued to treat his large cadre of addict patients in the manner he thought fit. Now under almost continual police surveillance, his name appeared repeatedly in the press, linked with drugs and scandal. As Delevingne observed, 'It has...been found impossible to proceed against him, but it is quite clear that he is prepared to give prescriptions for dangerous drugs to practically any person who asks for them.'[50] According to the authorities, he was supplying addict patients solely to keep them comfortable; he was willing to provide large doses on the basis of minimal face-to-face consultation, often using the postal service to distribute drugs or prescriptions, frequently at considerable geographical distances. For example, using the Royal Mail, he supplied patients in Glasgow and Paris. Although precise numbers are unobtainable, he had attracted large numbers of addicts to his West End practice; moreover, according to the Home Office and the police, these addicts were often of the underworld or vicious type. In addition, he chose to ignore advice and admonitions from the authorities, or 'played the system' to circumvent them, for instance, by signing the Home Office undertaking, which he clearly had no intention of fulfilling.

The Home Office, Rolleston and the Pursuit of Dr Connor

In the 1920s, the exploits of Dr Connor coincided with the work of the Departmental Committee on Morphine and Heroin Addiction; he was mentioned repeatedly at Committee meetings, and his was the first case listed in an appendix to the memorandum of evidence supplied to the Committee by Delevingne. Appearing twice, he was the prescriber in case

[47] *Times* 28 May 1923, p. 7; *Times* 2 June 1923, p. 9.

[48] *Aberdeen Press and Journal*, 2 June 1923, p. 8.

[49] TNA MEPO 3/1023, 'REX V. Samuel Grahame Connor: Particulars of cases coming to the notice of Police, taken from CID correspondence'.

[50] TNA MH 58/277, Appendix 1. Case 1.

numbers 5 and 25.[51] This document and its appended case summaries formed the centrepiece of the Home Office's evidence; the Committee was told that Connor had 'engaged the attention of the HO for many months…(and) the grounds for suspecting extensive abuse were overwhelming…'.[52]

The minutes record that 'the question of whether the Committee should invite Dr Connor…to give evidence was considered. The feeling of the Committee was in favour of his being called, but the final decision of the matter was postponed to a further meeting'. Delevingne responded to an inquiry on this point by stating that, 'We should see no objection to the Committee calling Dr Connor; in fact I was intending myself to propose that they should invite him to come'.[53] In the event, however, the invitation was not extended. This is unfortunate, for in all of the written material that has survived regarding Dr Connor and his scandalous prescribing, there is nothing to offer insight into his own perspective, excepting the highly formalised defences put to the courts and the GMC.

At last, just prior to the publication of the Departmental Committee's report in March 1926, the Home Office had a stroke of good fortune: in the course of inquiries into the case of a Miss Charlotte Young, Connor's records were inspected, and technical shortcomings were again identified. An unrepentant Glasgow addict in her 50s, Charlotte Young had been addicted for 20 years; she 'steadfastly declined to go into a home and is apparently prepared to take any steps to get the drug'.[54] Young had been prosecuted in Glasgow in 1922 for passing forged prescriptions. However, she was evidently a confident and independent woman, successful in business; according to Inspector Burmby of Scotland Yard, 'she was healthy in appearance, and was in many ways viewed as a respectable person. As to her drug consumption, the officer confessed that she thrived on it'.[55] In February 1924, the Home Office discovered that Connor too was prescribing for her, often by mailing supplies to Glasgow, and it was decided that this time an attempt should be made to prosecute him.

Despite pursuit across at least seven years of 'generous' prescribing, then, it was on technical record-keeping grounds that Dr Connor ended

[51] TNA MH 71/108, 'Memorandum prepared by the Home Office for the information of the Committee', cases 1, 5 and 25.

[52] Ibid. Case 1.

[53] TNA MH 71/108, 'Delevingne to Committee, 24 October 1924'.

[54] Ibid.

[55] *The Lancet* 207,5363 (1926) pp. 1146–50.

up in court. He had neglected to record three purchases of morphine from a manufacturing chemist, each for 50 grains, in his dangerous drugs register; there was a further count of failing to include the patient's address on one prescription—a total of four charges. Appearing at Marlborough Street police court on March 30, 1926, and with the Director of Public Prosecutions Sir Archibald Bodkin present in court for what was clearly viewed as a significant case, Connor pleaded guilty to the charges, arguing however that they were merely a matter of oversight.[56] Beneath the technical question, a fundamental struggle over the control of addiction was in progress.[57]

The stipendiary magistrate, Mr H. L. Cancellor, was greatly exercised by the physician's marginal and disreputable addict clientele. 'The defendant was not merely prescribing small quantities of drugs to people suffering from nervous diseases', he declared, 'but was making a practice of treating people who were addicted to drugs'.[58] It was confirmed, in addition, that many of these addict patients were 'known to the police'.[59] The type of addicts being treated by Connor was clearly a central issue.

Mr Cancellor then pointed out that Connor was something of a regulatory recidivist: 'He had had ample warnings, and had flagrantly disregarded them.'[60] Connor's prescribing was described by the prosecutor, who had no medical training, as 'excessive': in 1925, he had supplied Charlotte Young with 575 grains of morphine (over 37 grammes), while seeing her in person on only six occasions, the remaining doses being dispatched by post. Three of the four charges were for purchasing morphine without keeping a record; this was allowed when the drugs were for 'practice use': in these circumstances, the doctor would himself inject the patient in his consulting rooms, or the patient would administer it in his

[56] Marlborough Street police court was located in the centre of the West End and was the most celebrated of the capital's courts, excluding the Old Bailey. For an account of Marlborough Street court, see J. Lock, *Marlborough Street: The Story of a London Court* (London: Robert Hale, 1980).

[57] *Dundee Evening Telegraph*, 29 March 1926, p. 7. DPP Bodkin had followed the earlier development of the Connor case and gave evidence before the Rolleston Committee. See TNA MH 58/277, 'Summary of evidence of Sir Archibald Bodkin, KCB, Director of Public Prosecutions.' He also instructed the Home Office counsel at the GMC hearing. See *The Lancet* 207,5363, 1926. pp. 1146–50.

[58] *Daily Mail* 30 March 1926, p. 8.

[59] *The Times* 30 March 1926, p. 11.

[60] *Daily Mirror* 30 March 1926, p. 18.

presence. It was viewed as a technique that enabled the dishonest doctor to obtain drugs without leaving any record, and the implication in the courtroom was that this was Connor's motive.[61] The prosecution contention was that all of this constituted 'supplying' under the Act, and though no formal supply charge was made, the claim apparently made an impression on the magistrate.[62]

The question of fees was then raised, with Connor informing the court that his customary charge was one guinea per consultation, a sum which does not appear to have been exorbitant at this time. Nonetheless, proceedings did not go well. Once more the magistrate declaimed from the bench on the 'absolute' necessity that an erring medical man should be 'severely dealt with'; Dr Connor was, he said, 'making a practice of treating people who were addicted to drugs...the defendant had...been carrying on a practice most deleterious to his patients'. Accordingly, the doctor was found guilty, fined £200 and sentenced to six months' imprisonment. He was allowed bail and announced his intention to appeal. The appeal was largely successful, with the appeal judge concluding that Connor 'had been guilty of gross carelessness rather than wilful misconduct'.[63]

The original legal judgement was informed by discourses of improper clinical practice and unprofessional conduct, but there was a significant lacuna in the court's discussion. This was the fact that the Departmental Committee's report, published just weeks previously, had provided an authoritative justification for Connor's methods (aside from the record-keeping infringements, to which he admitted). This crucial fact did not feature in court. Appearing on appeal at the Old Bailey in April, Connor was successful in obtaining the remittal of the prison sentence; the fines were allowed to stand. On April 23, 1926, the customary notice appeared in *The London Gazette*, and Connor's authority under the Dangerous Drugs Acts to possess and supply drugs had been withdrawn. As a transgressive prescriber of narcotics, he was henceforth out of business.

[61] Doctors had to record supplies of dangerous drugs they purchased and supplied to their patients, 'but they did not have to record details of drugs they personally administered or which were taken by a patient in their presence'. H. B. Spear, *Heroin Addiction, Care and Control*, p. 11. This omission was removed by the 1971 Misuse of Drugs Act, Regulations, 1973.

[62] *British Medical Journal* 1,3406, (1926), pp. 677–678.

[63] *The Times* 17 April 1926, p. 9.

Addiction and the Struggle over Medical Authority

The next step for the Home Office was to act as the complainant in taking Connor's case to the Penal Cases Committee of the GMC. At a protracted hearing in June 1926, Connor faced charges of infamous conduct, and subsequent erasure from the medical register, over his treatment of drug addicts. Connor's methods were alleged by counsel representing the Home Office as falling outside the limits of bona fide medical practice. Both sides now invoked the regulations and ethics of the Rolleston Report. The use of dangerous drugs in treating addiction was, said Home Office counsel, permissible solely for its cure or attempted cure, or in minimum doses to enable an incurable addict to lead a useful life.[64] If a medical man became 'a mere purveyor of dangerous drugs for the gratification of an addict he ceased to be a person who was entitled to prescribe or use dangerous drugs, and the exemption provided under the Act no longer applied to him'.[65]

Connor's counsel too was quick to reference the 1926 Departmental Report, which laid down the principle that addiction was itself a disease, and described a class of persons for whom 'it might be necessary to continue to administer the drugs for a very long time if they were to lead useful and relatively normal lives'.[66] Dr Connor's treatment had been based on these principles, argued his legal representative, and his methods were quite within the law. Only a medical man could estimate the 'minimum dose' necessary, and the GMC could only judge Connor's motives in respect to his treatment of these patients by reference to his general character.

The GMC hearing ended with a year's probation, at the end of which Dr Connor was required to provide testimonial evidence from medical professionals and other 'persons of position' of his character, conduct and medical practice.

Returning to the GMC hearing in June 1927, Connor had prepared well. His clientele mirrored the heterogeneous metropolitan population that drew upon his services, cutting across the barriers of class and respectability. In addition to its drug addicts and sexual experimenters, Connor's practice comprised a considerable number of the great and the good, and

[64] *The Lancet* 207,5363, (1926), pp. 1147–1150.

[65] *British Medical Journal (Supplement)* 1,3414, (1926), pp. 213–215.

[66] Ibid.

these respectable patients and supporters provided testimonial evidence of his good character. They included J. A. R. Cairns, the police court magistrate; Sir Thomas Barlow, one of the 'bedside baronets'; and several other highly placed individuals; without doubt their testimony assisted Connor's case.

The GMC president informed the chamber that 'this…is the first case brought before the Council on a conviction under the Dangerous Drugs Act…'. The GMC had 'already issued a Warning Notice that not only convictions but contraventions which have not been the subject of convictions may be dealt with by the Council as offences which render a registered medical practitioner liable to have his name erased'.[67] This point is interesting: the GMC declared its intention to deal severely not only with breaches of the dangerous drugs legislation but with those that had not been before a court. Under section 29 of the Medical Act, practitioners contravening of the Dangerous Drugs Act and its regulations by abuse of their privileges might be erased from the medical register.

Despite its warning, the Council decided against any further sanctions against the doctor.[68] It was a decision that must have been disappointing to the Home Office, which had clearly hoped to have Connor entirely barred from medical practice.

The 1930s and the Script Doctor: The Consolidation of Transgressive Prescribing

In his sketch of these transgressive doctors, Spear locates Dr Arthur Edwin Tait as the next in line following the withdrawal of Connor's authority to possess and supply drugs.[69] Tait practised as a script doctor until 1939, when a record-keeping offence permitted the Home Secretary to withdraw his authority to possess and supply drugs. Following this, Tait's fortunes took a downward turn; during the 1940s he was to appear in court in connection with what appears to have been his new source of income—the receiving of stolen jewellery and associated ducking and diving. He received a prison sentence in 1948 and died the following year.

[67] *The Lancet* 207, 5363 (1926), p. 1150.
[68] Ibid.
[69] H. B. Spear, *Heroin Addiction, Care and Control,* p. 51.

Another figure that should be included in the late 1920s chronology is that of Dr Richard Starkie.[70] Starkie was a former Metropolitan Police surgeon who had been struck off the register in 1922 for practising abortion and turned his hand to supplying heroin in 1929 (i.e. while lacking the medical authority to do so).[71] Starkie had only two clients, a bogus major and an Italian princess, but prescribed large amounts to them and was in consequence sentenced to a year's imprisonment.[72]

The linkage of abortion with the transgressive supply of drugs is striking, and by no means consigned to the Starkie case; in Connor's example, following the withdrawal of his authority to supply drugs, he turned to abortion as an alternative way to make a living from medicine and practised very large numbers of 'illegal operations'. The Met described him as a 'notorious and clever abortionist...(who) may well be classified as the most systematic abortionist in London'.[73] The shared status of abortion and drugs as 'grey areas' for the medical profession is mirrored in their subcultural intertwining, and in their later shared designation as 'West End legal'.[74] State and professional regulatory agencies monitored the medical profession for infractions by disreputable doctors with regard to both, and it was in the 1930s that the establishment of transgressive prescribing or 'script doctoring' took hold as a sort of professional ghetto which some practitioners inhabited, and which often included abortion and the sympathetic treatment of problems related to homosexuality, venereal diseases and contraception. Some practitioners apparently entered and remained within this field as a matter of conscious decision. However, a number of material and structural changes underpinned and facilitated the consolidation of the transgressive prescriber. Amongst these were, in no assumed order of causal priority, the transformation of the Harley Street medical district and its impact on the medicine practised in the West End and inner London more widely, the advent of all-night pharmacies in this district and the presence of an opiate-consuming culture based in the capital.

[70] *Times* 3 December 1929, p. 11.

[71] *Times* 17 September 1921, p. 5.

[72] These were 'Major' Geoffrey Wilmer aka Melville and 'Mrs Melville', whose real name was Phoebe Aldo-Nordi.

[73] TNA MEPO 3/1023, 'Confidential Report respecting Dr Samuel Grahame Connor', 21 July 1937.

[74] See P. Ferris, *The Nameless: Abortion in Britain Today* (London: Pelican, 1967).

The Harley Street District

Harley Street, Wimpole Street and Welbeck Street were at the centre of an area of elite medicine that emerged in the mid-nineteenth century and expanded northward from the Cavendish Square end of Harley Street. Medical practice in the district 'differed significantly from what went on elsewhere'.[75] Initially, its resident doctors were the peers and neighbours of their upper-class patients, who were willing to pay for the 'bedside manner' at least as much for any claimed specialist knowledge. It was to the Harley Street area that morphine-dependent Brenda Dean Paul and her mother Irene went when their respective health problems drove them to enter to nursing homes, despite the family's relative poverty following the 1922 separation of Irene from her husband, the fifth baronet Sir Aubrey Dean Paul.[76] The women had a general practitioner based near their Chelsea home, but the reputation of Harley Street drew them to its specialists when pressed by serious medical need. In the 1920s, this continued to be an arrangement typical of the upper classes.

Nonetheless, by the mid-1930s, the character and reputation of the district was undergoing a series of transformations. As many of their wealthy patrons moved away from the West End to the London suburbs, the doctors followed them, often maintaining Harley Street consulting rooms while setting up house further from the centre. This migration freed up property, enabling other types of practitioners to move in, taking advantage of newly available lets, sublets and timeshares to occupy a space in the elite medical district that had previously been closed to them. As Humphrey points out, the street's approximately 200 medical addresses in 1904 had become 800 by 1938.[77] At the same time, an influx of foreign practitioners from the continent, many of whom were Jewish, some of them psychoanalysts, led to a perceived downgrading of the area's reputation, diluting the elite with newcomers of doubtful ethnic, social and cultural provenance, practising forms of treatment that existed at the limits of conventional medicine.[78]

[75] C. Humphrey, 'Place, Space and Reputation: The Changing Role of Harley Street in English Health Care' Social *Theory and Health* 2, 2 (2004), pp. 153–169.

[76] B. D. Paul, *My First Life: A biography* (London: Dent, 1935). Brenda Dean Paul is discussed in detail in Chap. 3 of this book.

[77] C. Humphrey, *The Changing Role of Harley Street*. p. 158.

[78] J. C. Adams, *Harley Street: A brief History with notes of nearby Regent's Park* (London: Royal Society of Medicine Press, 2008) p. 68.

While only a few of what came to be known as script doctors availed themselves of consulting rooms in the heart of the new, multi-tenancy medical district, the area's eclectic cocktail of medical practice, embracing both elite specialisms and marginal doctoring, soon pervaded the metropolis more generally. The ambivalence attaching itself to the capital's leading medical district reached beyond those few streets to practitioners in the inner London area, providing those who practised at the margins, such as the abortionists and script doctors, with a kind of cultural camouflage and permitting them to cater to their various clienteles. People would travel from all over the country to the West End of London—cosmopolitan and comparatively tolerant, fast moving and anonymous—for an abortion or a prescription for morphine.

The advent of 24-hour pharmacies was also conducive to making London the prescribing capital of the UK and the focus of the 1930s drug subculture. Boots had opened its 24-hour Piccadilly branch in the mid-1920s; by the 1930s, it had been joined in providing this all-night service by John Bell and Croyden in Wigmore Street, adjacent to the Harley Street medical district, and by Allen and Hanburys.[79] It is widely recognised that these pharmacies acted as points of communication and exchange for the opiate consumers of the 1960s; it is also highly probable that they served the same purposes for the earlier networks, though secure evidence of this has yet to emerge.[80]

Such a setting constituted the backdrop for the script doctor, who provided prescribing services to a growing network of morphine, heroin and cocaine consumers that had the ability to pay for the privilege. In the subsequent chapter, which focuses on the case of Brenda Dean Paul and the network of opiate consumers at whose centre she resided, the consolidation of the script doctor is clearly apparent. In the later 1930s and the Second World War years, a transition was visible in the pattern of medical practitioners providing services to the new, subcultural London addicts. This shift can be illustrated by examining those who prescribed for Paul in the early years of her addiction and comparing them with those of the later period. In the early 1930s, her physicians were a highly varied group, ranging from eminent practitioners whose bedside manners had won them

[79] Anon. 'Providing the capital with a 24-hour service', *Chemist & Druggist,* 202,4941 (1974) pp. 768–769.

[80] K. Leech, *Keep the Faith, Baby: A close-up of London's drop-outs* (London: S.P.C.K., 1973) p. 28.

royal patronage and a Harley Street address, like Dawson of Penn, through the ambivalent Mayfair physician Dr Frederick Stuart, who had also been involved in the Billie Carleton affair, to Dr Spira of Half Moon Street in Shepherd Market, whom the police viewed with great suspicion.[81] The important point is that these doctors varied greatly in social and professional status, in their attitudes toward the treatment of addiction and in their relationships with the regulatory authorities. At the close of the 1930s and during the Second World War, however, the situation had changed, and the type of practice favoured by the script doctors was more consistent in its operation. All those consulted by Paul at this point fitted more or less securely into the script doctor category; at best, they had uneasy relations with the regulators; the provision of the prescription lay at the heart of their method, treatment often being accompanied by little else; the prescriptions were what the Home Office regarded as 'generous' in their dosages, and grew more so with the passage of time; they drew relatively large numbers of addicts to their practices, and the authorities believed that they were motivated by the alleged pecuniary advantages of addiction treatment. The script doctor figure had become established in the medical landscape, albeit at the margins, where it was now a semi-permanent feature, while those who worked within it tended to be increasingly confined to and identified by the specifics of the role. Between the mid-1930s and the mid-1950s, Dr Tait, Dr Ripka, Dr Quinlan, Dr Sharp, Dr Swan, Dr Rourke, Dr Maguire, Dr Pinches, Dr Thompson, Dr Adler and Dr Freeman were all viewed by the Home Office as fully fledged script doctors.[82] Moreover, this list is not exhaustive, omitting some of the minor cases, nor does it include the infamous 'generous prescribers' of the second Brain Committee report who came later, such as Lady Isabella Frankau.[83]

[81] 'Brenda Paul Fit to be Liberated: Famous Doctors to be Called in Drug Case' *Daily Express* 9 March 1933, 3; Anon., 'Failure to Comply with Dangerous Drugs Regulations' *British Medical Journal* 2,3588 (1929), 694; TNA MEPO 3/2579, 'Copy of H. O. Minutes 583825/2 Brenda Dean Paul- Addict'.

[82] HO 45/18469, Lectures on Dangerous Drugs, 1940; TNA MEPO 3/1054, 'Supplies of large quantities of morphine by Dr. M.D. Ripka to Brian Dean Paul, drug addict, and brother of Brenda Dean Paul, 1936–1947.'; MEPO 3/2579, CID Memo, 6.11.1943; 'Drug Summons Dismissed' *Times* 9 September 1955, 5. Spear, H. B. & (ed) Mott, J. *Heroin Addiction, Care and Control: The British System*. London: Drugscope, 2002.

[83] MEPO 3/2579, Metropolitan Police Report—Regular Supplies 30.05.1963.

The Tribunal System and the GMC: Failure to Curtail Prescribing in the Quinlan Case

The 1926 Departmental Report had provided the Home Office with a specific mechanism for curtailing the operations of these injudicious prescribers prior to any intervention under criminal law; as we saw earlier, stopping such prescribing had represented what were often insuperable difficulties for the authorities. The mechanism devised by the Rolleston Committee was the medical tribunal. Under the 1926 Regulations, a medical tribunal could be appointed, and on its recommendation, the Home Secretary could withdraw from a practitioner the authority to possess and supply dangerous drugs. The Rolleston Committee had believed that such a mechanism could deal with the difficult problem of contested prescribing without the publicity that surrounded cases in the criminal justice system.[84] However, the complications of providing evidence to tribunals, which were unable to compel the attendance of witnesses, the fact that these witnesses were often addicts and thus considered unreliable, and the availability of alternative methods of dealing with doctor addicts and script doctors (i.e. the Home Office's preference for withdrawal of authority following prosecution under the dangerous drugs laws) meant that, on the UK mainland, tribunals were not utilised during the classic period of British drug regulation.[85]

However, there continued to be cases of practitioners whose prescribing style drew the concerned attention of the Home Office, yet who had committed no regulatory offences. Only the tribunal mechanism could offer a means of stopping transgressive prescribing in cases where no laws had been broken by the practitioner, and the decision not to use it had far reaching consequences. One such instance was that of Dr Gerald Quinlan of Maunsel Street SW1, a quiet thoroughfare close to the Houses of Parliament. In 1942, Dr Quinlan was prescribing for around two dozen of the best-known 'vicious' addicts in London, including Brenda Dean Paul and her brother Napier, along with Jean Baird and Freda Roberts; the Met wrote to the Home Office regarding Quinlan and 'the numerous

[84] *Departmental Committee on Morphine and Heroin Addiction: Report* (London: HMSO, 1926) Paras. 66–75.

[85] TNA HO 319/1, Inter-departmental Committee on Drug Addiction (Brain Committee): minutes of 1st, 2nd, 3rd and 4th meetings 1959; minutes of 1st and 2nd meetings 1960; matters arising from meetings; submission of report to Home Secretary.

drug addicts that are flocking around him'.[86,87] They believed Quinlan to be assisting Brenda Dean Paul in her attempts to evade arrest for 'double-scripting' by seeking refuge in a private nursing home. Paul had been obtaining supplies of heroin from both Quinlan and Dr Swan of Regent's Park Road NW1; Detective Sergeant Garrod, one of the Met's leading drugs officers during the Second World War years, had noted that 'both these doctors are well known to police and the Home Office as "script" doctors'.[88] Quinlan was, commented the Met, 'a person who cannot be trusted so far as his patients are concerned…and very little can be done about it'.[89]

Like other practitioners that followed, Quinlan was adept at remaining within the letter of the law, never giving the Home Office the opportunity to withdraw his authority to prescribe as had eventually been done in the instance of Dr Connor. With the tribunal system lying in neglect, the Drugs Branch looked once more to the disciplinary committee of the General Medical Council to curb Dr Quinlan's transgressive prescribing. According to the account offered by Spear, the Council was never very enthusiastic about taking on this role.[90] Nevertheless, under pressure from the Home Office, Quinlan was notified by the GMC that he would be required to appear before the disciplinary committee. He was to be charged with 'infamous conduct in a professional respect' as a result of his prescribing for known addicts 'other than for purposes of medical treatment'. As in most of these script doctor cases, no evidence remains to offer the physician's own perspective on his mode of addiction treatment.

In the event, Quinlan's appearance before the Council was repeatedly postponed, allowing him time to adjust his treatment methods in

[86] TNA MEPO 3/2579, 'CID Memorandum 16 October 1941'.

[87] Each of these addicts is discussed in Chaps. 3 and 5 of this work.

[88] TNA MEPO 3/2579, 'CID Memorandum 06 November 1943'.

[89] Ibid.

[90] H. B. Spear, *Heroin Addiction, Care and Control*, p. 54. Spear quotes an unreferenced letter from Heseltine, then GMC Registrar, stating that the Council would have preferred a legal case to be made against Quinlan under the DD Acts. Nonetheless, they would consider the use of professional criteria to bring Quinlan before the disciplinary committee on the grounds that 'he had sold large quantities of dangerous drugs to patients' at excessive rates, or frequent intervals, or otherwise than in bona fide treatment, and that knowing these patients were addicts he continued to do so 'to their moral and physical detriment'.

order to reduce both the number of addict patients and their dose levels; in these circumstances, the Home Office abandoned its plans, and in due course, the GMC ceased to pursue the case.[91] It was one of the first cases in which the regulatory regime proved itself quite unable to effectively intervene to curtail a form of addiction treatment it regarded as wholly unacceptable and as lying outside the spirit of the Acts framed by parliament. This inability would prove increasingly problematic to the Home Office as the 1950s and 1960s ushered in an expansion of the London opiate subculture, supported by a range of new prescribing doctors. By the 1950s, script doctors were aware that under the present laws, providing they kept within certain bounds—consisting largely of record-keeping requirements—they could not be prosecuted nor their prescribing otherwise impeded. Their numbers had grown, and the quantities of drugs supplied to addict patients were now in principle unlimited.

Reflecting on the Quinlan case in the course of the first Interdepartmental Committee on Drug Addiction in the late 1950s, the GMC stated that: 'In 1942, a difficult case arose which in the opinion of the Council illustrated the importance of maintaining and utilising, when the occasion arose, the machinery which had been provided (i.e. the tribunal devised for this purpose by Rolleston).'[92] In the light of the Quinlan case, reported the Council to the Home Office, it had 'unanimously decided that the Home Office should be urged, in any similar case in the future, to refer such a matter to a reference tribunal'.[93] However, no such referral was made during the period covered by this research. Instead, in circumstances in which a script doctor avoided breaking the law, he was in practice free to continue to make supplies of drugs available to his clientele. In consequence, script doctors provided the supply base for the white drug culture that for half a century co-existed with the British System; as will be illustrated in Chap. 3, this availability was a necessary but not sufficient condition for that subculture's emergence and development through subsequent decades.

[91] Ibid.

[92] TNA HO 319/1, Letter from Mr Pike Lees, GMC Registrar, 'Representations from the General Medical Council', 25 March 1960.

[93] Ibid.

Script Doctors and the Professionalisation of Medicine

Each element of the modernising, professionalising tendency in medicine, which began in the early and mid-nineteenth century, was countered by the methods and the dubious reputations of the script doctors.[94] The emphasis on the provision of the prescription, which gave these practitioners their Home Office title, ran counter to the increasing controls over the prescription pad that came with professionalisation, making them effective 'dealers in scripts and/or drugs' (moreover, some doctors continued to dispense their own drugs at this time).[95] While previously the property of the patient and capable of being filled repeatedly, use of the interwar prescription was now circumscribed, and in the case of dangerous drugs the prescriber was obliged to write upon it the instruction, 'Not to be repeated'. Running counter to this restrictive trend, the singular reliance of the script doctor on the prescription and the drugs for which it was the warrant, with little or no associated therapy, went directly against professionalised medicine as it was then being defined and was seen as reminiscent of the shopkeeper rather than the medical professional. The casual attitude toward the problem of dual and multiple prescribing exhibited by many of these practitioners further exacerbated this issue. The tendency to perform perfunctory examinations went hand in hand with this approach; the diagnostic skills that formed the centrepiece of a qualified doctor's arsenal were carelessly disregarded and reliance placed instead on the unevidenced claims of the patient. Furthermore, this style of practice came perilously close to the practitioner's tacit authorisation of self-medication by patients, another feature of the archaic medical culture that professionalisation had sought vigorously to suppress. The clustering of addicts around these doctors smacked of advertising; allegedly, at least one of them was accustomed to telephoning his addict clients to remind them that 'another prescription was due'.[96] It was also suspected that some practitioners were radically overcharging for their services, implicitly in

[94] I. Waddington, 'The professionalisation of medicine', *British Medical Journal* 301, 6754 (1990), pp. 688–690.

[95] See H. Whippell Gadd, 'The ownership of medical prescriptions', *The Lancet* 176, 4544 (1910), p. 1030.

[96] This was Dr Henry Irving Pinches; see TNA MH 58/565, 'Appendix Five, Section 1, case no. 2: Dr H. P.'

exchange for not pressing their patients sufficiently diligently in the direction of the residential 'cure'.

Appearing regularly in the national press and in the courts of law, transgressive prescribers acquired reputations that threatened the broader professional charisma of interwar medicine. As the prohibitionist German physician Pablo Wolff commented: 'the so-called "script doctors" ... have shown themselves to be entirely unworthy representatives of our profession.'[97]

The Anticipation of Harm Reduction Practices?

While these practitioners were a varied group, some of whom undoubtedly fell far short of the Hippocratic ideal, and were viewed nearly unanimously by the Home Office, the police and the institutions of the medical profession as thoroughly venal, in truth their role was more complex, and the ethical positions involved more ambivalent. Elements of their practice could be said to anticipate the later stance of the harm reduction approach to drug treatment. Currently controversial in some parts of the world and mainstreamed into the state treatment system in others, harm reduction does not demand of drug users that they abstain from illicit use but seeks rather to minimise the risks involved, including through the provision of legal doses of drugs and the setting up of low threshold services which are quick and easy to access. These were precisely the key features of the practice provided by the injudicious prescribers. Indeed, the kind of drug prescribing for which the 'British System' became widely known and lauded could be argued as best represented by the methods of those condemned as 'script doctors'. The popularity of these transgressive doctors amongst addicts may in itself suggest that more orthodox versions of the post-Rolleston prescribing system were resisted by some patients, who wanted long-term or indefinite supplies at high doses rather than moralising attempts to compel them to endure unwanted residential cures. On the other hand, as will become apparent in the course of this text, large numbers of medical practitioners were unenthusiastic about the maintenance style of prescribing, and would have much preferred addicts to be incarcerated. Whatever the intentions of the celebrated Rolleston Committee, being treated by practitioners who shared popular prejudices

[97] P. Wolff, 'Alcohol and Drug Addiction in Germany: Part 2- Drug Addiction' *British Journal of Inebriety* 30, 4 (1933), pp. 160–171.

against addicts was, in practice, unlikely to have been a therapeutic experience.

The 1930s saw the movement from isolated instances of transgressive practitioners from a mix of marginal professionals including the compassionate and the eccentric to form a group that catered consciously to the growing, yet still tiny, opiate-consuming culture. With the consolidation of the Home Office Drugs Branch and police drugs experts, the elements of the drugs dance and the symbolic war of which it was a part were now in place. The next two chapters explore these subcultural drug networks, while this chapter concludes with a table mapping out the primary script doctors of the interwar period. With one or two exceptions mentioned above, the records of those practitioners coming under the headings of compassionate and eccentric have not survived; consequently, the following listing represents the transgressive doctors that caused the greatest alarm at the Home Office (Table 2.1).

Table 2.1 Main script doctors, from the 1920s to the 1950s[a]

Name	*Practice address*	*Period of known transgressive practice*	*Well-known patients*	*Mechanism used to curtail prescribing*
Dr Reginald Nitch Smith	10 New Bond Street W1	1917		GMC disciplinary hearing—removed from medical register
Dr Samuel Grahame Connor	Dryden Chambers, Oxford Street W1	1919–1926		Authority to prescribe withdrawn after DD offence
Dr Richard Starkie	Oakley Square, NW1	1929	'Major' Geoffrey Wilmer, Phoebe Ruby Aldo-Nordi	Removed from register in 1921 following abortion case; imprisoned for DD offences in 1930
Dr Arthur Edwin Tait	52 Bryanston Street W1 (near Marble Arch)	1927–1939		Authority to prescribe withdrawn after DD offence
Dr John Joseph Hirschmann	127 Maida Vale, W9	1935–1936	Names n/k, but several	Authority to prescribe withdrawn after DD offence

(*continued*)

Table 2.1 (continued)

Name	*Practice address*	*Period of known transgressive practice*	*Well-known patients*	*Mechanism used to curtail prescribing*
Dr Henry Irving Pinches	4 Collingham Road, (Kensington) SW5	1938–1955	Brenda Dean Paul, Jean Baird, Patricia Mallory, Catherine Moore (aka Tozier)	None
Dr Gerald Quinlan	6 Maunsel St SW1	1939–1941	Brenda Dean Paul, Brian Dean Paul, Jean Baird	None (GMC disciplinary hearing aborted)
Dr J. E. Sharp	1 Oakley Street, SW3	1932–1945	Brenda Dean Paul, Anthea Carew, Jean Baird, Ann Mitchell	None
Dr Marks Ripka	158 Gower Street, WC; 78 George Street, Euston	1935–1953	Brian Dean Paul, Angela Wyndham-Wilson, Robert Clement	
Dr W. A. M. Swan	70 Regent's Park Road NW1	1942–1943	Brenda Dean Paul	None
Dr John Oni Akerele	Messina Avenue, Kilburn	1946–1947	Wilfred Cooper (aka Tony Ross), Bertie Jarrett	None
Dr O. S. Thompson	n/a—was formerly assistant to Dr Pinches	1955–n/k	Anthony John Curtis, Phil Seamen, Jeffrey Aggray, Helen Mandarin Taylor	None
Dr Adler		1955–n/k	Anthony John Curtis	

(*continued*)

Table 2.1 (continued)

Name	*Practice address*	*Period of known transgressive practice*	*Well-known patients*	*Mechanism used to curtail prescribing*
Dr Joseph Michael Rourke	Kensington Church Street, W8	1953–1960	Barry Ellis, Brenda Dean Paul, Brian Dean Paul, Jean Baird, Dickie Devere, Broderick Walker	None (failed DDA prosecution)
Dr Edward Arthur Maguire	Linden Gardens, W2 (assistant to Dr Rourke)	1946–1955	Barry Ellis, Broderick Walker	None
Dr Harry Freeman	231 Clapham Road, SW9	1951–1959	Brenda Dean Paul, Jean Baird[b]	None

[a]TNA MEPO 3/2579; TNA MEPO 3/1054; TNA MH 58/277; TNA MEPO 3/1023; TNA HO 45/24948

[b]The table deals with script doctors; this does not include those practitioners I have classed as 'compassionate' and 'eccentric' earlier in this chapter. This is partly because the focus of the text is on the script doctor, and partly owing to the Home Office's concentration on the transgressive practitioners, whose practices they sought to suppress and whose records have survived in greater number

n/k not known

CHAPTER 3

The Chelsea Network and White Drug Use in the 1930s

Introduction

This chapter turns from doctors who specialised in the prescribing of morphine, heroin and cocaine in interwar Britain to focus on those who were consuming these drugs for pleasure and entertainment and were regarded by the Home Office and the police as 'vicious addicts'. As the book explores the intertwining of the regulatory architecture with the illicit consumers it sought to manage, those injudicious prescribers discussed in Chap. 2 will continue to play a part here. Their everyday practice provided the ground on which the Rolleston project was articulated and made concrete.

With regard to the title of the book and this chapter, 'white drugs' was a contemporary term referring primarily to heroin, morphine and cocaine. These were the modern drugs, the crystalline salts and powders containing alkaloids extracted from psychoactive plants; medicinally, they enabled the measurement of the precise doses required for technologically advanced therapeutics.[1] The main 'brown drugs' were opium and hashish, or Indian hemp as the latter was usually known. Culturally, this nomenclature was highly complex; its main operation lay in the division between 'the raw and the cooked', the natural and the processed, and their related racial and colonial themes of, on the one hand, the 'brown'

[1] D. T. Courtwright, Forces *of Habit: Drugs and the Making of the Modern World* (Cambridge: Harvard University Press, 2001).

C. Hallam, *White Drug Cultures and Regulation in London, 1916–1960*, https://doi.org/10.1007/978-3-319-94770-9_3

oriental, native and inferior, and its European and American, civilised white counterpart.[2]

As described in Chap. 1, the established historical narrative of what Spear called the quiet times understood the narcotic landscape of 1930s Britain as populated almost entirely by a species of genteel, middle-aged and middle-class morphine addicts, while addict subculture was notable by its absence. [3,4] The drug users of the 1930s were supposed to be therapeutically addicted, compliant with the medical model which saw drug use as pathological, discreet about their usage and geographically and socially isolated from other addicts.[5] However, there now exists a considerable body of evidence, some of it newly available to academic research, that challenges this picture. It is my argument, based predominantly on these new sources, that an opiate subculture existed in London from at least the early 1930s. It is notable that this subculture was highly social in its drug use and contrasted with the isolated addicts of the historiographic orthodoxy. They took drugs in small groups, both in flats and houses and in the thoroughly extrovert settings of nightclubs and parties.

It is important to clarify at the outset that it is not my objective to engage in a technical sociological debate regarding what does and what does not constitute a 'real' subculture, and whether such an entity existed prior to the 1960s. The argument is, rather, a historical one, based on new research indicating that many of the attitudes and behaviours which have been associated with subcultural drug use could be found in the interwar years, particularly in London: for example, drug-focused hedonism, a sense of shared identity amongst nonmedical users of drugs, the public statement of use (expressed primarily in terms of style and conduct), the justification of drug use and so on. These were the elements by which the presence of a drug subculture was defined in the 1960s, and similar characteristics may be identified in the years between the two world wars. The quiet times were not, it seems, as quiet as has been supposed.

[2] This phrasing is borrowed from the cultural anthropologist Claude Levi Strauss. See C. Levi Strauss, *The Raw and the Cooked: Mythologiques Volume 1* (Chicago: University of Chicago, 1983).

[3] Chapter 1 explores the dominant social and historiographic account of what Spear called 'the quiet times' between 1930 and advent of the postwar drug subculture.

[4] H. B. Spear, 'The early years of Britain's drug situation in practice: up to the 1960s' in J. Strang & M. Gossop, *Heroin Addiction and the British System: Volume 1* (London and New York: Routledge, 2005) p. 21, *passim*.

[5] P. Bean, *The Social Control of Drugs* (London: Wiley Blackwell, 1968) p. 113.

Some of those who contended that no drug subculture existed claimed that this was because there were no repressive mechanisms to produce a sense of being outsiders or others to the mainstream culture: nothing, that is, for a subculture to define itself against.[6] In place of the hostile measures taken by the state in, for example, the USA, a humane and medicalised 'British System' was alleged to support the UK's opiate addicts, supplying them with drugs and enabling them to function as respectable members of British society.[7] However, while the UK's drug control arrangements certainly did ameliorate some of the suffering that those dependent on opiates experienced in the USA, the medical supply of opiates remained inextricably bound up with a systematic field of legal, administrative, social and cultural restrictions that enforced a sense of otherness amongst at least some addicts.[8] In addition, the system of treatment recommended by the Rolleston Committee was implemented in irregular and uneven ways.

The key documents in which this research is grounded belong to a batch of police files that richly detail the multiple cases of investigation, monitoring, arrest and prosecution of a young woman of aristocratic background between the beginning of the 1930s and the end of the 1950s.[9] Her name was Brenda Dean Paul. These records, which also cover some of Paul's 'associates', demonstrate clearly the field of repressions to which drug users were subjected in Britain, despite the medical elements of the control apparatus for which the country became (to some extent justly) celebrated by observers abroad.

There were two main subcultural networks using white drugs in 1930s London, each emerging from a distinct cultural context. The first was the Chelsea group, which was geographically centred in that West London district, formerly the heart of Edwardian Britain's artistic and bohemian community and still possessing a 'bohemian' reputation.[10] The Chelsea

[6] A. R. Lindesmith, 'The Argot of the Underworld Drug Addict', *Journal of Criminal Law and Criminology*, 2, 29 (1938) pp. 261–278.

[7] H. F. Judson, *Heroin Addiction in Britain: What Americans can learn from the English experience* (London and New York: Harcourt Brace, 1974).

[8] C. J. Acker, *Creating the American Junkie: Addiction Research in the Classic Era of Narcotic Control* (Baltimore: The Johns Hopkins University Press, 2002).

[9] TNA MEPO 3/2579, 'Brenda Dean Paul, Drug Addict: activities and associates' 1931–1963.

[10] J. White, *London in the 20th Century* (London: Vintage Books, 2008) pp. 16–17, *passim*. See also M. Wishart, High *Diver: An Autobiography* (London: Quartet Books, 1978) p. 7.

group crystallised out of literary and artistic modernism and the period's cafe society or 'smart bohemia'. It was made up of individuals and small sets from a mainly aristocratic and upper middle-class background, amongst whom baronet's daughter Brenda Dean Paul became the most celebrated and notorious figure. This network shared some of the characteristics of the 1960s subculture—hedonistic drug use, sexual experimentation, a bohemian rejection of industrial work culture and its routines. However, the group also differed from the 1960s subculture in important respects, including—most significantly—the prominent role played by women, especially young women. The second grouping was the West End network, consisting mainly of opiate users and emerging in the second half of the decade. It was based on the night-time economy of the West End and had strong links to the criminal underworlds of both London and Paris.

Both groups feature in the work of Bing Spear, especially in the volume edited by his collaborator Joy Mott.[11] However, they are mentioned only briefly, and Spear pays minimal attention to their social and cultural composition and context, both of which are critical for a historical understanding. The present chapter is culturally and socially focused and based on historical research carried out in relation to the first of these groups, the Chelsea network. It makes use of police files detailing the surveillance of Paul and her associates in the 1930s, alongside a disparate set of memoirs and biographies in which these individuals figure.

Cultural Conflict in Britain Between the Wars

Turning to the question of historical context, Christopher Lawrence and Ann K. Mayer quote Harold Perkin in regard to the 'halfway house' that the interwar period represented, in which the culture and discourses of Victorianism co-existed with those of modernism.[12] This co-existence was also an ongoing cultural conflict in which the ideas and language surrounding drugs and addiction were caught up and mobilised. This struggle animated the modernist and bohemian backdrop within which the Chelsea drug scene first appeared and was linked to much wider themes of national identity, modernity, sexuality and pleasure, in which drugs played a symbolic

[11] H. B. Spear, *Heroin Addiction, Care and Control, passim.*

[12] C. Lawrence, & A. K. Mayer, (eds.) *Regenerating England: Science, Medicine and Culture in Inter-War Britain* (Amsterdam: Editions Rodopi, 2000). Perkin, H. *The Rise of Professional Society: England since 1880* (Abingdon: Routledge, 1989).

role. Major William Coles of the Home Office Drugs Branch observed in the 1930s that the reason why drug use was practised on such a small scale in the UK was that it was 'not a characteristic of the British race to indulge in narcotic drugs'.[13] Coles went on to comment that the USA, by contrast, was composed of an amalgam of races, many of whom had shown a historical predilection for the use of opiates, and predisposed that country to the widespread drug consumption for which it was known.[14] It was one way in which the anxieties surrounding nonmedical drug use in Britain played into debates over the impact of American influence that were prominent during the interwar years. France too figured in these cultural battles. Home Secretary J. R. Clynes observed that, 'the general moral standards of most of the European countries, and particularly France, are lower than those obtaining in this country'; it was feared that the proposed building of a channel tunnel would permit the further entry into Britain of the white slave traffic, the drug traffic, pornography and gambling.[15,16]

By contrast, those advocating cultural modernism and the valorisation of pleasure viewed these social and artistic developments as new and liberating phenomena deriving from the continent, and France in particular.[17] Paul's autobiography notes the magnetism of Paris: 'I had friends in various sets or *mondes* in Paris and decided that the more artistic and Bohemian of these would provide the most likely entree into the mysterious underworld I sought....'[18] The text narrates how she encountered a heroin addict named Leo, who was sufficiently wealthy and well-connected to maintain his habit 'without being dependent on doctors, and with little risk of being involved in trouble with the police'. Watching fascinated as he prepared his heroin dose, she remarks, 'Here was the sort of thing I had indeed been looking for in Paris.'[19]

[13] Royal College of Physicians Archive: Royal College of Physicians Committee on Drug Addiction, 1938. 'Report of Discussion with Major W. H. Coles of the Home Office on February 22nd 1938'.

[14] D. Musto, *The American Disease: Origins of Narcotic Control* (Oxford: Oxford University Press, 1987).

[15] TNA HO 45/13708, Dangerous Drugs and Poisons: Some implications of proposed Channel Tunnel (1920–1930). 'Clynes to Prime Minister, 2 June 1930'.

[16] TNA HO 45/13708, 'The Earl of Crawford and Balcarres Called and Examined', pp. 1–2, n.d.

[17] M. J. Lancaster, *Brian Howard: Portrait of a Failure* (London: Timewell Press, 2005) p. 170.

[18] B. D. Paul, *My First Life*, p. 85.

[19] B. D. Paul, *My First Life*, pp. 87–88.

While the issue of race continued to play a prominent role in the cultural politics of drugs and addiction, in the early 1930s, drugs functioned as signifiers in conflicts around gender and the place of women, and over same-sex desire or 'perversion'. Sir Aubrey Dean Paul called at Scotland Yard in November 1931 to inform detectives of his anxiety that his daughter 'might become a confirmed drug taker and bring disgrace upon herself and her family'. Sir Aubrey explained that she was 'not living with him and she was not under his control'.[20] Large numbers of the Chelsea network were women, many of them divorced and/or living apart from parental control, and several of the most prominent bisexual or lesbian. There was a great deal of ambivalence in British culture regarding the place of women, especially young women, who had recently obtained the vote; these drug-using women were in one respect a part of the generalised problem of the 'modern girl', and in another, they lived way beyond the narcotic and sexual limits of what the mainstream culture was prepared to accommodate.[21]

Changes to the Composition of Britain's Upper Classes

If it was implicated in the problematic relationships of gender and sexuality, the advent of this new group of addicts was in addition linked to changes in the social structure and culture of Britain's elite classes. In the 1920s and 1930s, the term 'society' as recorded in the national press referred not to the concept of the social totality as used by sociologists but to the publicly displayed social activities of the upper classes, which underwent far-reaching changes in the early decades of the twentieth century.[22]

The land-owning nineteenth-century aristocracy's social activities were based around the London Season, a structured calendar of social events (the state opening of parliament, the presentation of debutantes at court, the Mayfair balls, the Henley Regatta, Cowes, etc.) that 'brought together the great governing families of Britain, partly for pleasure and display, partly for political entertaining...and partly so that marriage partners

[20] TNA MEPO 3/2579, CID Memorandum 18 November 1931.

[21] L. A. Hall, *Sex, Gender and Social Change in Britain since 1880* (Basingstoke & London: Macmillan Press, 2000), p. 122.

[22] P. Balfour, *The Society Racket: A critical survey of modern life* (London: Long, 1933).

might be vetted and selected'.[23] The Season was an essentially ritualised performance of the articulation of political and social power. From the late Victorian period, the aristocracy became increasingly merged with an international (especially American) plutocracy for which wealth, glamour and celebrity counted much more than patrician lineage. A new type of press, focused on personality and image and initiated by the arrival on the scene of the *Daily Mail*, reported on the lifestyles of these 'smart sets'.[24]

Bohemia too, which had emerged in France as a subculture of opposition to the bourgeois order, reflected transformations in modern urban life, as the boundary marking off the elite classes and bohemia became porous and unstable.[25] According to art historian Andrew Stephenson, in bohemian spaces such as nightclubs, 'the social tone was much higher' during these decades. There were apache dances at Ciro's smart West End nightclub, cabarets at London's hotels and restaurants.[26] Such imagery, which before the First World War had signified a 'racy avant-garde bohemianism – daring tango dances, rough criminal gangs, outcast subcultural types and vital American jazz', had now become absorbed into parts of the entertainment mainstream. Stephenson comments that 'these passionate dances, sensational cabarets, racy music and underworld figures still carried the frisson of excitement that such imagined identifications represented as a way of shaping and configuring modern identities and testing society's sexual and racial limits'.[27] Such themes and images provided a symbolic means of representing identities as cultural and social insurgents.

Out of a merging of the smart set and the new bohemia came what the newspapers called the 'bright young people' (BYP).[28] This group, which

[23] D. Cannadine, *The Decline and Fall of the British Aristocracy* (London: Papermac, 1996), p. 342.

[24] A. Bingham, *Gender, Modernity and the Popular Press in Interwar Britain* (Oxford: Oxford University Press, 2004), pp. 22–34. See also S. Gundle, *Glamour: A History* (Oxford: Oxford University Press, 2008), pp. 140–144.

[25] E. Wilson, *Bohemians: The Glamorous Outcasts* (London: Tauris Parke, 2003).

[26] 'Apaches' were French gangsters; the term was widely used at this time.

[27] A. Stephenson, 'New ways of modern bohemia: Edward Burra in London, Paris, Marseilles and Harlem'. *Tate Papers*, no. 19, Spring 2013. http://www.tate.org.uk/research/publications/tate-papers/19/new-ways-of-modern-bohemia-edward-burra-in-london-paris-marseilles-and-harlem, accessed 12 November 2015.

[28] D. J. Taylor, *Bright Young People: The Rise and Fall of a Generation: 1918–1940* (London: Chatto & Windus, 2007). See also P. Horn, *Flappers: The real lives of British women in the era of The Great Gatsby* (Stroud: Amberley, 2013), pp. 33–57; P. Horn, *Country House Society:*

came to be seen as representing the youth of the aftermath, featured heavily in the popular press from the mid-1920s, and was known for its extravagant all-night parties, hedonism, jazz, racial and sexual experimentation and heavy consumption of cocktails. Many individuals who found themselves at the heart of the Chelsea drug scene had previously been part of the BYP.

There is a certain irony in the fact that it was the records of investigation and surveillance left behind by the Metropolitan Police that enable us to trace the crystallisation of an opiate-consuming subculture out of these new forms of smart bohemia in 1920s and 1930s London. Police surveillance of Brenda Dean Paul began in early 1931, tracing her cab journeys around the iconic West End spaces of bohemia and the BYP: the Eiffel Tower hotel and restaurant in Percy Street, W1, a celebrated social centre for modernist writers and artists prior to the outbreak of the First World War, colonised in the interwar years by the smart set; the Gargoyle Club—situated in Dean Street, Soho, and founded in 1925—which was erroneously referred to in police memoranda as the 'Girl Guides' Club'; the smart and fashionable Coliseum Theatre in St Martin's Lane; The Ring in Blackfriars Road, a famous boxing venue. Detectives were also in pursuit during Paul's visits to the Blue Lantern in Ham Yard, Soho, perhaps the key nightclub for the most 'raffish' elements of the BYP, and to Uncle's, around the corner in Albemarle Street.[29,30,31] These spaces supported a loosely defined cultural movement that was complex and heterogeneous,

The private lives of England's upper class after the First World War (Stroud: Amberley, 2013), pp. 191–211; S. Gundle, *Glamour: A History* (Oxford: Oxford University Press, 2008), pp. 153–161; C. Dyhouse, *Girl Trouble: Panic and Progress in the History of Young Women* (London: Zed Books, 2013), pp. 71–104; D. Fowler, *Youth Culture in Modern Britain, c. 1920–1970: From Ivory Tower to Global Movement- A New History* (Basingstoke: Palgrave Macmillan, 2008), pp. 59–71. G. Playfair *Six Studies in Hypocrisy* (London: Secker & Warburg, 1969).

[29] P. Brooker, *Bohemia in London: The Social Scene of Early Modernism* (Basingstoke: Palgrave Macmillan, 2007), pp. 123–131. See also V. King, *The Weeping and the Laughter: An Autobiography* (London: MacDonald and Jane's, 1976). pp. 89–91; C. Ross, *Twenties London: A City in the Jazz Age* (London: Philip Wilson, 2003) pp. 38–40, and V. Nicholson, *Among the Bohemians: Experiments in Living 1900–1939* (London: Penguin, 2003), pp. 268–9.

[30] C. Ross, *Twenties London: A City in the Jazz Age* (London: Philip Wilson, 2003), p. 38.

[31] M. Luke, *David Tennant and the Gargoyle Years* (London: Weidenfeld and Nicolson, 1991).

but united around the ideas it drew from modernism and its opposition to the old conservative order of the Victorian and Edwardian periods.

Conceptual Tools and Further Characteristics of Drug Subcultures

In thinking about the ways in which drug subcultures operated during the period covered by this and the following chapter, I employ a loose tripartite schematic. The individuals involved were first of all linked in terms of the *set*, a concept I take from the popular linguistic usage of the time: for example, 'Brenda Dean Paul and her set' refers to the group of people socially closest to Paul in the 1930s. The second conceptual term is the *network*, which is a larger structure made up of multiple related sets. In interwar Chelsea, the drug scene formed as a network through the interweaving and overlapping of sets and the individuals who were part of them. Finally, at the highest conceptual level, there was the *subculture*, which encompassed the totality of intermediate sets and networks. It should be noted that it is not my intention to elaborate a fully developed theoretical model; rather, these should be viewed as practical conceptual tools that permit the thinking through of a field of relationships operating across those who consumed, accessed and exchanged drugs.

It is not possible to accurately estimate the numbers of those involved in the Chelsea network. They were engaged in a type of hidden behaviour, which was illegal and carried relatively heavy penalties, and only those who were either prosecuted and whose cases were covered by the press, or who appear in surviving police files, or feature in memoirs and biographies from the period, remain accessible to historians.

Moreover, the boundaries of these networks were neither fixed nor clearly demarcated; there were those at the centre whose lives were powerfully focused on drugs, others at the margins who consumed in ways that would today be called recreational. Individuals and sets also varied the intensity of their engagement over time and according to circumstance. Traces of some of the key figures from these groups may be retrieved from the various historical materials; I shall provide biographical sketches of some of these in the course of exploring the functioning of the network.

The Functioning of the Chelsea Network: Doctors

The primary business of a drug subculture was the consumption of drugs, which implied, in turn, the accessing, exchanging and selling of drugs. Bound up with this was the important matter of generating and sharing drug knowledge, the practical know-how associated with obtaining and using drugs, avoiding interdiction and so on. The Chelsea network was supplied primarily from medical sources. Consequently, information about and access to doctors was at a premium, and possession of such know-how an imperative piece of subcultural capital. Its possession raised one's status in the network.

Acquiring drugs was not a simple matter of visiting one's local physician. It was true that, in accordance with the regulations obtaining under the Dangerous Drugs Acts, any doctor could in theory be approached for a prescription for drugs with which to treat addiction. In practice, however, some doctors were much more amenable than others: as we saw in the previous chapter, certain practitioners were ready to supply large and frequent doses, to post prescriptions and drugs at a distance, and did not bother to obtain a second opinion concerning treatment involving a prescription (a second opinion was recommended by the Rolleston Committee). They exercised minimal pressure on patients to undertake institutional cures and would accept the referrals of addict friends. The most useful practitioners from the perspective of the vicious subculture were the script doctors, a metropolitan medical specialism that became increasingly entrenched as the 1930s progressed, as discussed in the previous chapter.

The addict who appeared to have possessed the most extensive know-how when it came to identifying and accessing suitable prescribers was Brenda Dean Paul. Paul is usually regarded as the centre around which the Chelsea white drug scene revolved. It is difficult, if possible at all, to distinguish the extent to which this central position is merely a historiographic artefact, a reflection of the greater attention paid to her by both contemporary and subsequent writers, including the press and the police. When Paul's drug use first appeared in the newspapers, she was already a figure bathed in fame and glamour, and the case attracted a great deal of comment.[32] At the same time, she was undoubtedly a charismatic individual whose example could be highly influential to others.

[32] *Daily Mirror* 7 December 1931, p. 6; *Daily Express* 7 December 1931, p. 7; *Times* 7 December 1931, p. 7.

Brenda Irene Isabelle Frances Theresa Dean Paul (1907–1959) was born in Kensington, London.[33] Her parents were Sir Aubrey Dean Paul, fifth baronet, and Irene Regina Wieniawska, who became Lady Dean Paul upon their marriage in 1901.[34] Irene was the daughter of Henryk Wieniawski, a celebrated Polish violinist and composer; she had followed her father's profession as a composer and musician, working under the pseudonym Poldowski.[35] Brenda inherited from her mother a wide network of friends in the UK and on the continent ('almost a brotherhood'), which provided her with an early entrance to high bohemian circles in which drug use was relatively commonplace.[36,37] She had a short career as an actress in the early 1920s, after which she travelled extensively, visiting metropolitan centres such as New York, Berlin and Paris.[38] Paul was one of the original and most prominent participants in the BYP, and it was this phase of her life that inaugurated her status as a glamorous celebrity.

Her first prosecution came in December 1931, when she appeared at Marlborough Street police court accused of multiple scripting offences (obtaining drugs from several doctors at once) and prescription forgery (she had altered the amount on a morphine prescription). Frederick Mead the magistrate, still sitting in his 80s, ordered Paul to be bound over for three years, conditional upon her entering a residential home for drug treatment. She appeared in court again the following year, when the Tower Bridge magistrate Morgan Griffith Jones sent her to prison for six months, a sentence overturned on appeal in the subsequent month by the London Sessions court, which once more imposed a residential cure condition, and

[33] For previous discussions of Brenda Dean Paul, see R. Davenport-Hines, *The Pursuit of Oblivion: A Global History of Narcotics 1500–2000* (London: Weidenfeld & Nicholson, 2001), pp. 294–297; V. Berridge, *Demons: Our changing attitudes to alcohol, tobacco and drugs* (Oxford: Oxford University Press, 2013), pp. 162–163; H. B. Spear, *Heroin Addiction, Care and Control*, p. 52; J. Savage, *Teenage: The Creation of Youth 1875–1945* (London: Pimlico, 2008), pp. 235–237, p. 245, p. 247.

[34] P. Hoare, 'Paul, Brenda Irene Isabelle Frances Theresa Dean (1907–1959)', *Oxford Dictionary of National Biography*, (Oxford: Oxford University Press, 2004) http://www.oxforddnb.com/view/article/64889, accessed 14 Dec 2014.

[35] D. Mooney, 'Poldowski Rediscovered', *Dublin Institute of Technology* http://arrow.dit.ie/aaconmusart/4/ Accessed 10.03.2016.

[36] B. Dean Paul, *My First Life: A biography* (London: Dent, 1935), pp. 85–86. See also J. Kavanagh, *Secret Muses: The Life of Frederick Ashton* (London: Faber & Faber, 1996), p. 70.

[37] V. Berridge, 'The Origins of the English Drug "Scene" 1890–1930' *Medical History*, 32, (1988), pp. 51–64.

[38] Paul, *My First Life* p. 81, *passim*.

two sureties of £250 each.[39] In 1943, Paul served a six-month sentence for unlawful possession of heroin, again as a consequence of multiple scripting. Her life continued to feature such clashes with the authorities, her drug use continuing until her death from natural causes just prior to the dawn of the 1960s.[40]

Paul was an expert at identifying and ranking medical practitioners according to their use as suppliers of drugs. The fact that several Chelsea addicts were patients of Dr Sharp of Oakley Street, Chelsea, was not a coincidence or an accident of geography but a function of the subcultural network.[41] Of course, there is no way to prove this, but it is extremely likely that other addicts, some of whom lived faraway, were referred to Dr Sharp by Paul. Indeed, script doctors depended upon the efficient operation of the network in order to practise their disreputable specialism, which required the attendance of several patients. These doctors relied on the network 'grapevine'. The Chelsea network acted as a system of relays, permitting the circulation of this recondite subcultural knowledge, referral and supply.

Dr Sharp later became a full-blown script doctor. The police observed that 'addicts have suddenly commenced to flock round this doctor and in all probability others will follow, the reason being…that he charges less than other doctors for his prescriptions'.[42] Officers believed that 'before long he will be assuming the role of Dr Gerald Quinlan, whose activities in the past as a "script" doctor are so well known'.[43] Such knowledge of Sharp's bargain prescription prices would certainly have been passed around the addict network.

Paul, possessor of an encyclopaedic store of practical knowledge of London's medical men and their prescribing preferences, could, in addition, arrange introductions for her friends and acquaintances to the most desirable script doctors even if she was not herself a patient; in the postwar era, for example, she arranged for her 'associate', the prostitute, Kathleen Moore, to see Dr Henry Pinches (a script doctor well known to the police and one of Paul's former prescribers) in order to obtain a prescription for cocaine.[44]

[39] Sureties are funds held by the court as a guarantee of the defendant's good behaviour. One of the sureties in this case was put up by Gwen Plunket Greene, mother of David Plunket Greene. Paul, *My First Life*, pp. 233–241.

[40] *Daily Express* 27 July 1959, p. 1.

[41] For more on Dr Sharp, see Chap. 2.

[42] TNA MEPO 3/2579, CID Memorandum D.S. Garrod, 13 October 1945.

[43] Ibid.

[44] MEPO 3/2579, CID Memorandum, 20 November 1951.

The police were doubly suspicious of some of these medical practitioners. Abortion was at this point illegal, and the women of the Chelsea network were adjudged to be sufficiently morally dubious to seek out the services of these marginal doctors to obtain abortions. Police reports noted euphemistically that Paul 'occasionally has to enter Nursing Homes for treatment of abdominal complaints'.[45] Detectives on surveillance duties even investigated her visit to the Devonshire Street home of the eminently respectable Mr Harold Chapple, senior obstetrician and gynaecologist at Guy's Hospital.[46]

Some of the locations to which officers pursued Paul and her associates no doubt appeared to lend weight to their suspicions. There were regular journeys to the Shepherd Market area of Mayfair, known as both a queer subcultural enclave and domain in which sexual services could be purchased. In Half Moon Street, where Reggie de Veulle had lived, the surgeon Edward 'Teddy' Sugden had his consulting rooms.[47] An abortionist and provider of contraception, Sugden later achieved notoriety through his involvement in the Profumo affair.[48] However, in the 1930s the area was already a hub for subcultures and marginal medical services.

With reference to the supply of drugs, the Met suspected Dr J. J. Spira of injudicious prescribing from his consulting rooms in Half Moon Street. Spira was well known to the Dean Paul family, and had prescribed morphine for both Brenda and her mother Irene, though treatment for the latter was unrelated to addiction.[49] Following inquiries into Spira's prescribing and a visit from the Regional Medical Officer, Arthur Anderson of the Home Office Drugs Branch wrote that 'Dr Spira's answers are so roundabout and his general attitude so unsatisfactory that I am by no means satisfied that that what he tells us is the exact truth'. Nonetheless, no proof could be found, and no further action was taken with regard to Spira.[50]

[45] TNA MEPO 3/2579, D.I. Barker, CID Memorandum 16 February 1931.

[46] TNA MEPO 3/2579, D.I. Inspector Barker, CID Memorandum 23 May 1931.

[47] Reginald de Veulle was a dressmaker and a drug user who was alleged to have supplied Billie Carleton with cocaine. See Kohn, *Dope Girls*, pp. 91–95, *passim*. For de Veulle in Half Moon Street, see M. Houlbrook, *Queer London: Perils and Pleasures in the Sexual Metropolis, 1918–1957*. (London: University of Chicago Press, 2005), pp. 113–114.

[48] R. Davenport-Hines, 'Sugden, Edward Charles' (1902–1982) *Oxford Dictionary of National Biography*, (Oxford: Oxford University Press, 2004).

[49] TNA MEPO 3/2579, D.I. Barker, CID Memorandum 16 February 1931.

[50] TNA MEPO 3/2579, Copy of Home Office minute 585,825/2.

One of Paul's closest friends in the early 1930s was Anthea Rosemary Carew (1906–1960), who was born in Chelsea. Anthea was the daughter of Henry Gamble, the Dean of Exeter, and, in a lavish society wedding in 1928, married *The Times* sports journalist Dudley Carew at Exeter Cathedral. The marriage, wrote Dudley Carew later, had an 'air of unreality' about it and lasted only months.[51] The Met noted in early 1931 that Anthea Carew was 'regarded as a "Bohemian" type and is friendly with Miss Dean Paul. She is a heavy drinker'.[52] Shortly afterwards they discovered that Carew was also a morphine addict. She was prosecuted twice in 1932, both cases involving Paul. Firstly, Carew was attempting to purchase cocaine on credit from a French countess who was staying briefly in London; the cocaine was for Paul who was suffering from opiate withdrawal sickness and found that cocaine was one of the few substances that helped.[53] Secondly, Carew sent Paul some morphine from Exeter to London by Royal Mail, only to find the parcel intercepted by the police, who were conducting surveillance on both women. In the event, Anthea Carew was fined one shilling and bound over on condition she underwent a residential cure at Mowbray House, a nursing home near her mother in Exeter. In the later 1930s, she moved to Yorkshire, though she continued to use morphine when visiting London, obtaining supplies from the well-known script doctor, Dr Sharp of Chelsea.[54]

During the early phase of the investigation of Paul and Carew, the Home Office sought to identify medical men who might be supplying them with morphine. Anthea Carew told police that when she was in Devon, Dr Valentine of Appledore 'supplies her with all the morphine she wants'. Likewise, Dr Sharp provided drugs more or less on request. Neither of these practitioners gave prescriptions but, she alleged, supplied her with drugs directly.[55] Such a manoeuvre made it more difficult for the police to trace drug supplies, and the Home Office was put on the alert by this information. Once again, however, they were unable to produce sufficient evidence to take action.

In addition to the script doctors sought out by the Chelsea network, there were other medical men who were reluctant to prescribe drugs or, if

[51] D. Carew, *A Fragment of Friendship: Evelyn Waugh as a young man* (London: Everest Books, 1974) p. 81.

[52] MEPO 3/2579, CID Memorandum 16 February 1931.

[53] The 'countess case', as it was termed in the popular newspapers, is discussed below.

[54] TNA MEPO 3/2579, CID Memorandum 13 October 1945.

[55] TNA MEPO 3/2579, 583,825/21.

they did prescribe, rapidly reduced doses and pressurised addicts to undertake residential cures. It was those practitioners who adopted a stricter approach to the supply of drugs who appear to have met with official approval. Dr Viney, a Kensington general practitioner who was amongst the earliest to treat Paul, told her that she would have to undergo a complete cure if she wished to retain him as her medical advisor. The Regional Medical Officer who saw Viney in regard to Paul declared himself 'very favourably impressed' by the practitioner, concluding that 'Miss Dean Paul has been fortunate in her choice of a doctor who is able in his treatment of her addiction to combine kindness with firmness'.[56]

Leonie Fester (1896–1949) was another Chelsea network addict; she had recently divorced her second husband and was living on the Kings Road with her daughter Carmen.[57] Fester was forced by her doctor to reduce her dose. She had repeated offences for multi-scripting, and like numerous other subcultural addicts of the period, she was allowed probation on the grounds that she underwent a residential cure.[58] This provides us with another reminder of the legal architecture that functioned in cooperation with the more familiar prescribing elements, and significantly modified addicts' experience of the British System. While the Rolleston-inspired regulations did facilitate the prescribing of drugs on a long-term or even permanent basis (depending on the circumstances), it was a matter for the individual medical practitioner to decide on what was the appropriate treatment in each case, and views on addiction and its treatment varied considerably. Mainstream patients would have little idea of doctors' views on such a question.

The Countess Case: London, Paris and Transnational Drug Networks

A related function of the network was the sharing of knowledge of, and access to, illicit supplies of drugs. An example in which these operations may be traced is represented by the so-called countess case, which featured

[56] TNA MEPO 3/2579, Report of Dr Selby R.M.O., 8 June 1931. Paul also speaks highly of Dr Viney in her autobiography: see Paul, *My First Life* pp. 177–179.

[57] TNA MEPO 3/1673, Statement of Mrs Leonie Fester 2 June 1932.

[58] *Yorkshire Post* 31 January 1933, p. 5. Leonie Fester was also suspected by the police of trafficking offences; see MEPO 3/2579, CID Memorandum 16 January 1933. See also 'Dangerous Drugs Acts', *Chemist & Druggist*, 118, 2765 (1933) p. 108.

in British and international newspapers in 1932. Before narrating this case, I will discuss one more key protagonist.

Brian Kenneth Napier Dean Paul (1904–1972) was Brenda's brother and was to be the last of the baronetcy. Described by Scotland Yard as a 'young man of effeminate habits and manners, who does not appear to follow any occupation', Napper, as he was generally known, was another participant in the BYP scene and was very close to his sister, sharing her taste for alcohol and opiates.[59] In 1937, despite his homosexuality, Napper married Muriel Weigall, widow of the well-known Egyptologist and sister of comedienne Beatrice Lillie.[60,61] An enthusiastic cross-dresser, for much of his addict career, Napper seems to have supported himself by pilfering and other petty crimes, though in the early 1930s he occasionally described himself as an 'interior designer', a fashionable occupation in the period.[62] Curiously enough, Napper was never prosecuted for drugs offences and seems to have evaded a warrant for his arrest for taxi bilking in 1939.[63] A police officer, speaking in court, told the magistrate that Brian Dean Paul 'was seen at Marylebone this morning and warned to attend. I think it is useless adjourning the case. He has defied everyone'.[64] On his father's death in 1961, Napper inherited the family title and was listed in police records as Sir Brian Kenneth Dean Paul.

Briefly, the details of the countess case were as follows. Marie Lanfranc (1893–n/k), who upon her 1910 marriage had become the Comtesse de Flammerecourt, was a convicted drug trafficker in her home city of Paris, a kilogramme of unspecified drugs having been found in her home in 1930. She resided in Rue Chambiges, a smart thoroughfare in the city centre. The Paris police were very concerned with her morals, stating that she was 'an adventuress capable of anything to obtain money'. In addition, she was considered predatory and sexually degenerate: 'her life is very

[59] MEPO 3/2579 CID, Memorandum 16 February 1931.

[60] Ken Leech recalled meeting 'Napper' Dean Paul in the Golden Lion, a well-known gay pub in 1970s Soho. Personal Communication, 2013.

[61] J. Hankey, *A Passion for Egypt: Arthur Weigall, Tutankhamun and the 'Curse of the Pharaohs'* (London: Tauris Parke Paperbacks, 2007).

[62] A. Lycett, *Dylan Thomas: A New Life* (London: Phoenix, 2004), pp. 214–215.

[63] Taxi 'bilking' was a vernacular term for absconding without paying one's cab fare. It was used by both the police and the public.

[64] *Times* 1 November 1939, p. 3. Brian and Brenda Dean Paul's offences were discussed at the same hearing.

animated; she frequents night halls and night clubs in Paris with a view to meeting an occasional lover…'.[65]

In August 1932, she was enjoying a short stay in London, allegedly to sell cocaine. The visit came to the attention of the Met, who, with the permission of the manager at the Hotel Somerset in Orchard Street, W1, searched her room and found a small packet of cocaine in a drawer.[66] While the search was underway, Brenda, Napper and Anthea Carew arrived at the hotel in pursuit of the countess; all three were arrested, suspected of conspiring to procure drugs. The countess was arrested on suspicion of unlawful possession.

The initial contact between the countess and the Dean Paul set took the form of a series of letters delivered by messenger and written by Anthea Carew, in which she explained obliquely that Brenda was suffering from withdrawal sickness and that 'the only thing that will get her through is Coc'.[67] Paul too weighed in with a letter, which was intended to be understood only by those 'in the know'—though its coded references sound innocent to twenty-first-century ears: 'You have said that if she (Anthea) wishes she can yet have some hats. She wishes to spend another £20 because the hats are so pretty.'[68]It appears from this series of letters that Carew had been introduced or referred to de Flammerecourt by a mutual contact, who is known only as 'Terence'. This is, once more, the network functioning, for it transpired that Carew was in fact asking for drugs on credit and using 'Terence' as a reference of her willingness and ability to pay. The mysterious Terence had indeed provided both the introduction and reference for Anthea Carew, each of which indicated that the countess placed considerable trust in him. In the event, the appearance of Detective Sergeant Griffey of the Yard had undone the process, and Anthea, for all her efforts on behalf of Brenda, faced prosecution for attempting to procure cocaine.[69]

The identity of the 'Terence' featured in this correspondence is a matter of speculation; whoever he was, he appears to have had good contacts with

[65] TNA MEPO 3/2579, Translation of report from Paris, 15 October 1932.

[66] The Met heard of de Flammerecourt's presence in London through a Dr Ripman, who was then treating another addict. Ripman was reluctant to disclose his own source of information, but notified Griffey at Scotland Yard about the countess. TNA MEPO 3/2579 DS Griffey CID Memorandum, 4 August 1932.

[67] TNA MEPO 3/2579, Copy of letter marked No. 1.

[68] TNA MEPO 3/2579, Copy of letter marked No. 2.

[69] MEPO 3/2579, CID Memorandum, D. S. Griffey, 4 August 1932.

the Paris drug scene. Indeed, the Chelsea network in general was rich in contacts in that city, which seems by some distance to have been the major source of illicit white drugs circulating in London. At the centre of the Parisienne bohemian scene in 1920s and 1930s was the writer, artist and film-maker Jean Cocteau (1889–1963). Cocteau published his famous novel *Les Enfants Terribles* in 1929, and the hotel rooms he occupied in Paris, Villefranche and elsewhere became the sites of pilgrimages for youth from much of Europe and the USA. Cocteau was an opium smoker for most of his life and introduced numerous others to the practice.[70]

Among those who knew Cocteau well, and were at the heart of a set within the Chelsea network, was Jose Antonio de Gandarillas (1887–1970), or 'Tony' as he was known to his friends. Gandarillas was a wealthy Chilean diplomat who lived in London and Paris and had a house in Cheyne Walk, Chelsea. He almost certainly taught the English painter Christopher Wood (1901–1930) to smoke opium, and in the 1920s, the two journeyed to Smyrna in Turkey, a major centre of opium production. Gandarillas was not a trafficker but probably supplied his friends, as he usually had the best opium.[71] During the Second World War when border restrictions were tightened, he was apprehended for bringing the drug into England in the Chilean Embassy's baggage. He was 'addicted to the inhalation of opium', said the Home Office, which allowed him thereafter to obtain opium legally.[72] These connections undoubtedly enabled the movement of drugs from Paris to London. Again, it is impossible to quantify the traffic; while the Comtesse de Flammerecourt's visit to London became public due to a court case, most visits and exchanges did not.

To summarise, in relation to illicit drugs, networks provided drugs, knowledge, introductions, mutual recognition and subcultural 'references' that could offer access to the former elements, as well as extend lines of credit between people who did not directly know one another. This is a very different matter to a simple collection of unrelated individuals, and quite distinct from the relationships obtaining between medically compliant, respectable addicts who are alleged to have exclusively populated the drugs map of 1930s Britain.

[70] F. Steegmuller, *Cocteau: A Biography* (London: Constable, 1986), pp. 342–343.

[71] S. Faulks, *The Fatal Englishman: Three Short Lives* (London: Vintage, 1997), p. 27.

[72] TNA HO 45/24948, Annual Report of the Home Office Dangerous Drugs Branch for 1940.

Drug Use in the Chelsea Network

The group was known for its use of opiates and, to a lesser extent, cocaine. It appears that during the early years of the 1930s, there were sets with preferences for different opiate drugs: for example, Brenda Dean Paul, Anthea Carew and Napper Dean favoured morphine, while Ruth Baldwin and Olivia Wyndham were heroin consumers. Ruth Baldwin (1905–1937) was born in America. Though few details survive, she features in the margins of several memoirs from the period and was known for her prodigious intake of heroin, cocaine and alcohol. She is alleged to have 'turned her kitchen into a bar' and lived with the well-known lesbian heiress and speedboat racer Joe Carstairs at Mulberry Walk in Chelsea.[73] She was part of the set that included the painter Edward Burra, along with society portrait photographer Barbara Ker-Seymour. Ruth died of a suspected overdose at a Chelsea party in 1937, while her friends listened to a boxing match in the next room.[74,75]

Olivia Wyndham (1897–1967) was another high bohemian lesbian who was an originator of the BYP. Her younger half-brother Francis Wyndham left an account of Olivia in his *roman a clef* novelette *Mrs Henderson*, writing that 'Brenda Dean Paul by her persuasively poised example led her on to experiment with heroin and cocaine'.[76] In truth, however, while she may have been inspired in part by Paul's example, she did much more than 'experiment' with these drugs: she was a long-term, intensive user, as well as an alcoholic. A passionate enemy of racism, Wyndham began a relationship with the black American actress Edna Thomas while the latter was in London, following her back to New York where Thomas had set up a successful salon that was a centre of the Harlem renaissance. Despite Olivia's habit of buying drugs on the streets of Harlem and returning to the apartment with assorted addicts, pimps and prostitutes, theirs was a lifelong relationship.[77]

Dolly Wilde (1895–1941), niece of Oscar, was another member of this lesbian addict set. She was simultaneously an element in the Paris literary salon of Natalie Barney but sought strenuously, if ultimately unsuccessfully,

[73] K. Summerscale, *The Queen of Whale Cay* (London: Fourth Estate, 1997), pp. 78–79.
[74] *Times (Royal Edition)* 2 September 1937, 'Deaths', p. 1.
[75] J. Stevenson, *Edward Burra: Twentieth-Century Eye* (London: Pimlico, 2008), p. 216.
[76] F. Wyndham, *Mrs Henderson* (New York: Moyer Bell, 1985), p. 60.
[77] J. Stevenson, *Twentieth-Century Eye*, p. 214.

to keep these two identities apart.[78] Much of the overlap between different subcultural networks, though, came from individuals participating in culturally adjacent sets, for example, the high proportion of lesbians and queer men in the Chelsea network. Literary historian Susan Zieger notes the close relationship between sexuality and addiction, in terms of both pathologising discourses and overlapping urban subcultures.[79] Notably, the West End network, differing here from its Chelsea counterpart, was to have its primary overlap with different subcultural groupings: criminals and those working in the West End's commercial sex trade.

Entry into the Chelsea Network

How was it that some of those belonging to smart bohemian circles like the BYP, which featured occasional drug use, went on to form a subcultural network in which the consumption of opiate drugs was the core component? This question can be answered in part by the series of intoxications in which these groups indulged, broadly moving through the use of alcohol, proprietary medicines containing opiates and other substances, to the nonmedical use of semi-licit or illicit supplies of morphine and cocaine.

One of the first characteristics of the 1930s Chelsea sets to be noted by police surveillance was the intensifying use of 'pick-me-ups'. Detectives followed up their pursuit of Paul and Carew's taxicab journeys to chemist shops by interviewing many of those they had visited, and were informed by several pharmacists that Paul was 'a frequent purchaser of pick-me-ups'.[80] Harry Walker, an early member of Paul's set and manager of Soho's Gargoyle Club,[81] was 'indebted to a chemist in Knightsbridge to the extent of over £50 which has been mainly incurred by the purchase of "pick-me-ups"'.[82] Such reports indicate an intensive consumption of these substances, which remained available from pharmacies without prescription. Their potency had been limited by the 1920 Dangerous Drugs Act to 0.2 per cent in the case of morphine and 0.1 per cent for cocaine (and

[78] J. Schenkar, *Truly Wilde: The Unsettling Story of Dolly Wilde, Oscar's Unusual Niece* (London: Virago, 2000), p. 130, *passim*.

[79] S. Zieger, *Inventing the Addict*, pp. 159.

[80] TNA MEPO 3/2579, Inspector Barker, CID Memorandum 16 February 1931.

[81] M. Luke, *David Tennant and the Gargoyle Years* (London: Weidenfeld and Nicolson, 1991), pp. 34, 36, *passim*.

[82] TNA MEPO 3/2579, Inspector Barker, CID Memorandum 23 May 1931.

heroin, until 1925 when its inclusion in patent medicines was prohibited).[83] Despite the reduction in active alkaloid content, these preparations had their uses. It is probable that recourse to such remedies began as a method of ameliorating the after-effects of alcohol, which had been consumed in large quantities by practically all of the BYP during the 1920s; police reports state that Paul, Carew, Harry Walker and Miles Cory were all heavy drinkers.[84]

Cory was a wealthy former army officer, who was at the heart of the network in 1930. He was allegedly an alcoholic and had at first injected Paul with morphine with the objective of reducing her alcohol intake. Subsequently, he provided supplies 'for her own use by personal injection'.[85] In addition, the Home Office learned that when Paul visited her family home at Appledore in Devon around this time, she had obtained sufficient morphine from Cory to see her through her absence from London. Miles Cory is a plausible contender for the role of Brenda's supplier. He was wealthy and well-connected, and probably used morphine himself, either to withdraw from alcohol or to better handle its after-effects. As noted in an unpublished PhD thesis by Holly Crossen-White, army officers and retired army officers were strongly linked to drug use and supply in the early twentieth century.[86] Whatever its origins, Brenda's addiction went back much further than she had confessed to the police: Dr Thomas Creighton, who was a house physician at the Park Lane Hotel in 1928 when he was consulted by Brenda on an unrelated matter, stated that he had been aware of her morphine addiction then.[87]

So, the main pathway into regular consumption of opiates for those in the Chelsea network appears to have been linked to the use of alcohol. Heavy drinking was a key element of the hedonism of the smart set in the 1920s and was informed by styles and attitudes of refusal toward both US prohibition and the UK's onerous restrictions on drinking within the night-time economy.[88] Alcohol was then supplemented by recourse to

[83] *Departmental Committee on Morphine and Heroin Addiction: Report* (London: HMSO, 1926), para. 90.

[84] TNA MEPO 3/2579, Inspector Barker, CID Memorandum 16 February 1931.

[85] TNA MEPO 3/2579, Home Office Memo, Godfrey Street, 30 January 1931.

[86] H. L. Crossen-White, *Drug related activity in the United Kingdom of Great Britain and Ireland between 1900 and 1922: What evidence can be found through systematic searches of The Times Digital Archive?* (Unpublished PhD Thesis, Bournemouth 2012), *passim*.

[87] TNA MEPO 3/2579, Statement of Dr Thomas Creighton n.d.

[88] E. Mannin, *Young in the Twenties: A Chapter of Autobiography* (London: Hutchinson, 1971), p. 32.

'pick-me-ups', which trailed a long history of uses linked to 'sobering up' and could also be employed to tide addicts over during periods when more potent drugs were unobtainable, or to taper off during attempts at abstinence.

The step from alcohol and pick-me-ups to the use of controlled drugs was a relatively small one for those in the aristocracy and upper middle classes; consumption of opiates was considered acceptable amongst elements of the elite, an attitude which persisted despite the passage of the dangerous drugs laws.[89] Moreover, the aristocracy was used to getting its way in its transactions with professionals, and doctors were no exception.[90] Following the imposition of legal restrictions on drugs, the medical profession became the most readily available source of supplies. The upper classes found it easy to source drugs from one or more doctors—Paul was eventually prosecuted by an exasperated Home Office for obtaining drugs from several doctors simultaneously, some known to the Dean Paul family, at least one an injudicious prescriber, others attached as house physicians to the smartest hotels in central London. These were the doctors who catered to the addicted elite at the beginning of the 1930s and made the step to regular opiate use a simpler one than it might otherwise have been.

Cultural themes, of course, played a key role in the transition from the bright young people into the Chelsea drug network. Many of these networks overlapped, but an interesting clue to the linkage is offered by writer and journalist Dudley Carew, who partnered Anthea (nee Gamble) Carew in a short-lived marriage in 1928. Carew sought to defend the BYP from the condescension of posterity, reflecting in the austere years after the Second World War:

> If it is a virtue…to care little for self, to take no heed of consequences, to be utter and extreme in the risks of friendship and of love, to have no need for personal and material advantage, to give recklessly of money and emotion, and to care, in some secret and unadvertised way, for the line and form of

[89] P. Ziegler, *Diana Cooper* (London: Hamish Hamilton, 1981), pp. 54–55. See also P. Horn, *Country House Society: The private lives of England's upper class after the First World War* (Stroud: Amberley, 2013), pp. 21–22; and, J. Fox, *White Mischief* (London: Vintage, 1998), passim.

[90] M. Pugh, *'We Danced All Night': A Social History of Britain Between the Wars* (London: Vintage Books, 2009), p. 45.

> beauty, then the "lost generation" can take some credit it was careful never to give itself.[91]

If the description fits the BYP, the Chelsea network took this imperative of recklessness further still and was, perhaps, the first generation of 'beautiful losers'.

Subcultural Perspectives on Drug Use

Relatively little has survived to tell us how this early subculture understood itself. Such texts as are available were constructed by authorities such as the police and the medical profession, who often had little or no understanding of the views and attitudes of these marginal people. Moreover, though many were well-connected with the press and generated a considerable quantity of text for newspapers, they were severely constrained in terms of what could and could not be said in this public setting. Paul's autobiography, for example, for which she was remunerated by the *Sunday Dispatch* and which was at least partly ghost-written, or at best co-produced with a journalist, tended at times to reiterate the standard tropes of the didactic drug story.

Paul and others did sometimes speak out regarding the ineffective nature of the dangerous drugs laws and associated policies. 'The laws regarding drugs have been made for the fools', she wrote.[92] The novelist Mary Butts, an opium smoker who had been an associate of occultist and self-proclaimed 'drug-fiend' Aleister Crowley in the 1920s and later a heroin addict and friend of Cocteau, made in her journals some prescient remarks regarding the unforeseen health effects of a repressive drug control system: 'Opium is dear, the supply uncertain, therefore people are reduced to re-cooking the dross, distilling the once-cooked dross, drinking it in coffee. Thus poisoning their insides, which moderate smoking would have affected very little. So much for restrictive legislation', she wrote.[93,94]

[91] D. Carew, *The House is Gone: A Personal Retrospect* (London: Robert Hale, 1949), p. 12.

[92] Paul, *My First Life*, p. 86.

[93] Aleister Crowley, *Diary of a Drug Fiend* San Francisco, Weiser Books, 1979. (First published 1922).

[94] N. Blondel, *The Journals of Mary Butts: Henry McBride Series in Modernism and Modernity* (New Haven: Yale University Press, 2003), p. 272.

One of the most interesting expressions of the subcultural views then obtaining occurred in 1932, when Mr Morgan Griffith Jones, magistrate at Tower Bridge police court who had just remanded Paul in custody and later sentenced her to six months' imprisonment, received a postcard from an unknown source.[95,96] Partly a tirade against Mr Morgan Griffith Jones, the 'arch fiend devil monster', the postcard also contains elements of discourse that defended and supported drug use. The court's 'treatment of a suffering woman is another instance of the sub-animal nature of the English', it declared, employing the 'sub-animal' adjective because the writer had initially termed the magistrate an 'animal', and then retracted the description: 'animals show sympathy with suffering'. The writer continues: 'morphine is a product of nature's wild flowers – the Poppy – nature is feminine and "men" like you do all you can to cut women off from their Divine Mother Nature'. The author argues that they do this by denying women access to the soothing remedies that feminine nature provides, despite that fact that 'millions use these remedies'. The postcard closes by criticising the priorities of the police, who 'instead of tracking down thieves…stalk suffering women who have done no harm to anyone!'.[97] Though this text is brief and somewhat garbled, it hints at a potentially valuable account of the views that must have circulated in the 1930s opiate subculture—how widely it is impossible to know, though the stated positions resemble those of thinkers such as Mary Butts. Essentially, it situates the consumption of opiates in terms of a kind of eco-feminism and argues that their use is both natural and therapeutic. Moreover, it associates Englishness with the repression of pleasure and emotion, a repression which underpins the dangerous drugs laws.

Others in the Chelsea group appeared to view the use of drugs more as a form of highly sophisticated entertainment. Brian Howard (1905–1958) came from a Jewish middle-class background and was a champion of modernism in art and literature at Eton and Oxford in the 1920s. Another erstwhile BYP, he was a flamboyant homosexual whose intellectual brilliance was read by his contemporaries as a sign of great literary promise. However, Howard's gifts were eventually directed into his everyday life

[95] *Daily Mirror* 23 August 1932, p. 5; *Times* 23 August 1932, p. 7.

[96] TNA MEPO 3/2579, Memorandum, Kennington Road Police to Home Office, 3 September 1932.

[97] TNA MEPO 3/2579, Anonymous postcard to Mr Griffith Jones, Tower Bridge Police Court, 31 August 1932.

and relationships, and his biography was (arguably somewhat harshly) entitled *Portrait of a Failure*.[98] Like many in the network, he was a heavy drinker and was in the 1930s engaged in the regular use of drugs, though not an addict. Following a trip to Germany, he was one of the first to take seriously the impending threat of the Nazis. In the postwar years, he led the peripatetic existence of an exile and became dependent on the use of heroin and other opiates.

Speaking with the writer Christopher Isherwood in 1935, Howard vividly explained that '*cocaine* gathered like a knot in the chest and was like ozone, while *heroin* spreads like a stone-flower from the stomach to the legs and arms', and *hashish* was like toffee and made you feel 'like the gateway to hell'.[99] Isherwood remarked that during this encounter, Howard was consuming cocaine with 'ostentatious sniffs', which again points to the subcultural characteristic of flaunting one's forbidden tastes and behaviour. Typical of the Chelsea network, he was a full participant in the overlapping subcultures of drugs and homosexuality.

If Brenda Dean Paul was a charismatic instance of drug use, Howard was too, and there were others. David Plunket Greene (1904–1941) was an example: six feet seven inches tall and an accomplished jazz pianist, 'more than anyone else he was representative of the age of jazz that shook Oxford in the twenties'.[100] Greene was a heroin addict and was remembered as an immensely attractive and fashionable dandy by his contemporaries. During the Second World War, he drowned in Shearwater Lake on the Longleat estate.[101] These magnetic figures are mentioned—and there are others that could be—to counteract the historiographic tendency to view Brenda Dean Paul as the hub of the network who drew all the others into her orbit.

The Chelsea network mostly elected to inject their drugs. This choice may have been made partly on grounds of pharmaceutical efficiency or medical experience but was also connected to the symbolic character of the hypodermic needle and syringe, and through this to its subcultural function as an indicator of social and cultural identity. Sociologist Dick

[98] M. J. Lancaster, Brian *Howard: Portrait of a Failure* (London: Timewell Press, 2005).

[99] M. J. Lancaster, *Brian Howard: Portrait of a Failure*, p. 216.

[100] M. Davie, (ed.) (1995) *The Diaries of Evelyn Waugh* (London: Phoenix, 1995), p. 800, quoting D. Fielding, (1954) *Mercury Presides* (London: Eyre and Spottiswoode, 1954). On the early jazz scene in Britain, see: C. Parsonage *The Evolution of Jazz in Britain, 1880–1935* (Aldershot: Ashgate, 2005).

[101] D. Fielding, *Mercury Presides* (London: Eyre and Spottiswoode, 1954), p. 195.

Hebdige famously explored the ways in which objects can signal subcultural identity and opposition to the dominant culture; his classic text begins with an account of French homosexual writer Jean Genet, who employed a tube of Vaseline to 'proclaim his homosexuality to the world', a mundane object which, within his social and historical context would, 'by its mere presence…be able to exasperate all the police in the world'.[102] The key point of Hebdige's work is that objects such as clothes, hairstyles, cosmetics, dances and so on can communicate cultural meanings. These meanings are, it must be added, historically contingent; in the interwar period, the group explored in this research expressed a form of revolt, not through any philosophical or political programme but through new styles of life and forms of consumption.[103]

Public Injection and Subcultural Belonging

In the 1920s, young women's short skirts, cropped hair, the use of cosmetics and cigarette smoking transgressed the social codes surrounding gender roles and femininity.[104] To inject drugs in public, however, represented a still more socially and culturally transgressive act. It remained strongly linked to the disruption of the roles and expectations associated with gender (doctors were almost exclusively male and the institutions of the profession a bastion of patriarchal power) and suborned the rational authority of medical professionals who had campaigned to restrict the syringe to exclusively medical use. In keeping with the disruption of codes proposed by Hebdige as the identifying mark of subculture, it transferred the act of injection out of the clinical domain into the world of entertainment and pleasure, where according to medical discourse it emphatically did not belong.

Several members of the Chelsea group would sometimes inject themselves in public—often at social gatherings. Paul occasionally practised this dramatic conduct, as remarked by her friend the British painter Michael

[102] R. Hebdige, *Subculture: The Meaning of Style*, p. 2.

[103] Cf. M. Kohn, (2001) *Dope girls*, p. 6.

[104] C. Dyhouse, *Girl Trouble: Panic and Progress in the History of Young Women* (London: Zed Books, 2013), p. 77. See also P. Tinkler, *Smoke Signals: Women, smoking and visual culture* (Oxford: Berg, 2006), pp. 84–93, *passim*; C. Horwood, *Keeping Up Appearances: Fashion and Class Between the Wars* (Stroud: The History Press, 2011), pp. 163, 167, 141–144, *passim*; C. Breward, *Fashion* (Oxford: Oxford University Press, 2003), pp. 220–222.

Wishart. Wishart wrote that he grew accustomed to witnessing Brenda injecting herself 'in a restaurant, produc(ing) from her handbag a hypodermic syringe of heroin, which she filled from a vase of flowers on the table…'.[105] Dolly Wilde was also known to behave in this spectacular fashion, 'as in the London dinner party during which she casually injected herself in full view…'.[106] Freda Roberts (1911–1967), a leading figure in the West End network until the prosecution of its main suppliers in the late 1930s, meanwhile went so far as to inject herself through her woollen skirt as she attended a marriage ceremony.[107]

Despite the solitary reputation of opiate use, such practices confirmed the fundamentally social nature of vicious addiction, which was recognised by the police and courts, who reiterated the importance of removing addicts from their network of addict friends and associates in order to produce a cure. Both Paul and Carew were subjected to such measures as part of their probation conditions. 'Clearly Miss Paul must be removed from her present bad companions', observed the Director of Public Prosecutions office in 1932.[108] Similarly, Carew's defence counsel was quick to stress in court that by sending her to her mother's care, she would be 'not be in London but in Exeter, where the influences were quite different'. Any visitors to the home would, he added, be vetted by her medical attendant.[109]

These drug cases were in addition attended by members of the network, and the courts became a theatre of symbolic conflict over both modern women and drug use, as well as (in Paul's case) an occasion of public notoriety and celebrity.[110] The newspapers regularly noted the presence in court of 'fashionably dressed women' and the 'excited rush of a number of young men to gain admission'.[111,112]

[105] M. Wishart, *High Diver: An Autobiography* (London: Quartet Books, 1978), p. 124.

[106] J. Schenkar, *Truly Wilde*, pp. 107–108, 130.

[107] A. Ashley with D. Thompson, *The First Lady* (London: John Blake, 2006), pp. 74–75. 'The registrar looked up, blinked and carried on', reports Ashley.

[108] TNA MEPO 3/2579, Memorandum from Director of Public Prosecutions, 12 April 1932.

[109] *Daily Express* 10 September 1932, p. 7.

[110] L. Bland, *Modern Women on Trial: Sexual Transgression in the Age of the Flapper* (Manchester: Manchester University Press, 2013), pp. 55–101, *passim*.

[111] *Daily Mirror* 12 November 1932, p. 16.

[112] *Western Daily Press* 6 September 1932, p. 5.

Drug Subcultures in the 1930s: A Road Less Travelled?

The advent of these networks came some 20–30 years earlier than the timing accorded to them in the pre-existing historiographic timeline of subcultural drug use in Britain. They shared many characteristics with their 1960s counterparts but nonetheless differed in significant ways. Importantly, they were much more feminised, and bore a family resemblance to the postmodern eco-feminisms that emerged in the wake of the 1960s counter-culture. The Chelsea network represents a route that the drug subculture might have taken in the postwar era, had not the North American version, with its emphasis on a masculine rejection of domesticity and often coupled with homophobia, achieved the predominant position in the discourses surrounding illicit drug use.

CHAPTER 4

Heroin and the West End Life, c.1935–c.1938

Introduction

During the second half of the 1930s, another subcultural, drug-using network appeared in London. It bore both similarities to and differences from the Chelsea group discussed in the previous chapter. In terms of class, though there was some aristocratic involvement, the West End network was more heterogeneous than its Chelsea counterpart; participants came predominantly from the middle classes but were also drawn from across the spectrum of Britain's class structure. In addition, they appear to have been younger on average than the Chelsea group. The disparities between the two were, however, most apparent in terms of culture: the West End network was not made up of individuals whose drug use began in high bohemia, nor (for the most part) do their names appear in the memoirs of interwar art or literature. Instead, the traces they left in the historical record were few or none, and those that did make their textual mark did so only via the press reporting of court cases.

Like the Chelsea addicts, though, this group emerged out of a broader, pre-existing subculture; but rather than artistic, literary and sexual bohemia, it crystallised from the night-time economy of London's West End—from the clubs and bottle parties that formed the marginal economy of the capital's pleasure district. The type of social existence that was supported by this grey area of economic activity is referred to here as the 'West End life'. The network shared much with Chelsea's bohemianism—for example, hedonism, antipathy to the workaday world, a libertarian sexual

C. Hallam, *White Drug Cultures and Regulation in London, 1916–1960*, https://doi.org/10.1007/978-3-319-94770-9_4

ethic—but was distinctive in its consumerism and its aspirational lifestyle. It was also much more tightly interwoven with the criminal underworld and the sex industry, and deeply involved in the trafficking and supply of drugs.

This grouping has been the subject of very little historical research. It is discussed in just over half a page of text by former Home Office dangerous drugs inspector 'Bing' Spear, whose information had probably been passed on to him by Frank Thornton.[1] Thornton first joined the temporary Home Office formation working under the Defence of the Realm Act regulations and the Dangerous Drugs Act of 1920, which officially became the Home Office Drugs Branch in 1933. He was a member of some of the same clubs as the leading figures in this network and, according to Spear, knew some of them well; he took over the leadership of the Branch in 1943.[2] Spear also hints that Thornton was drawn to the nightclub world for reasons that went beyond the purely professional, but does not elaborate on his remark.[3] More recently, historian James H. Mills has examined various members of this network, his account focusing on the cannabis use practised by some of its members and on the regulatory responses to their illicit entrepreneurial activities.[4] Other than the work of Spear, his police contemporary Detective Sergeant George Lyle, and Mills' historical monograph on cannabis consumption and control in the UK, nothing has been written about the group.[5,6] Moreover, relatively little remains by way

[1] H. B. Spear, *Heroin Addiction Care and Control*, p. 52.

[2] H. B. Spear, *Heroin Addiction care and control*, p. 59.

[3] The peripatetic style of policing London's West End, which involved the acquiring of experiential knowledge of the demimonde, was one which a number of police memoirists claimed to have adopted and which equipped its practitioners with skills that could not be gained in less direct ways. As former Metropolitan Police Superintendent Inspector Robert Fabian informs us: 'For twenty-eight years the West End has been my office table and work-bench.' On this 'office table', Fabian claimed to possess a range of key contacts and informants. He adds: 'I did not make the acquaintance of these people from the *Police Gazette*. I got to know them in the haunts and dives where they spent most of their time.' R. Fabian, *London After Dark: An intimate record of night life in London, and a selection of crime stories from the casebook of Ex-Superintendent Robert Fabian* (Kingswood, Surrey: Naldrett, 1954) pp. 10–11.

[4] J. H. Mills, *Cannabis Nation: Control and Consumption in Britain, 1928–2008* (Oxford: Oxford University Press, 2012) pp. 20–24.

[5] G. Lyle, 'Dangerous Drug Traffic in London' *British Journal of Addiction* 50,1 (1953) pp. 47–55.

[6] H. B. Spear, 'The early years of Britain's drug situation in practice: up to the 1960s' in J. Strang & M. Gossop, *Heroin Addiction and the British System: Volume 1: Origins and Evolution* (Routledge, London and New York, 2005).

of archival resources; some police records of the clubs with which the group was associated have survived, and a short selection of documents relating to the arrest and prosecution of Gerald O'Brien, its leading figure, for heroin offences.[7] Alongside these sources, there are contemporary newspaper accounts that provide important pointers into the operation of the network and the lifestyles of its most prominent figures.

It is my contention that there remains considerably more to be said about this network and that it contributes not only to a revision of the accepted narrative of interwar opiate use and addiction but tells us much about the links between drug use and the cultural geography of the West End of London, links which lasted throughout the twentieth century. The West End network represented a second drug subcultural network, which, though it possessed little in the way of any ideological elaboration of its lifestyle, practised a mode of life that was itself expressive and comprised a set of transgressions in relation to the often-implicit social codes of 1930s Britain. Once again, it was the symbolic power of drugs that incited the regulatory and representational responses characteristic of the era. Anxieties surrounding drugs were in this case closely tied to the perception that Mayfair, amongst the capital's most prestigious districts of upper-class residence and sociability, was facing a flood of social and cultural disorder—drugs, prostitution, gambling, crime and moral decay—coming from the adjacent district of Soho. I will begin by examining the functioning of the network and providing a short biographical sketch of its major players.

West End Network: Composition and Leading Players

At the centre of this network was Gerald Edward Mary O'Brien (1910–1954). O'Brien's name points to his ethnic background in catholic Ireland. He was a nephew of Desmond FitzGerald, who fought for the Irish nationalist cause in the Easter Rising of 1916, taking part in the firefight at the Dublin Post Office and later going on to become Defence Minister in the government of the Irish Free State.[8] Desmond was the

[7] TNA MEPO 3/1056, 'G.E. O'Brien: sentenced to six months for possessing dangerous drugs at Lewes', 1937; TNA MEPO 2/4487, 'Illegal sales of liquor at West End night bar: imprisonment for defendant already serving sentence for drug offences', 1937; TNA MEPO 3/1038, 'League of Nations Advisory Committee on traffic in opium and other dangerous drugs: quarterly summaries from July 1934–1939', Case no. 964.

[8] *Daily Express* 8 July 1937, p. 9.

father of Garrett FitzGerald, who was the Taoiseach in the 1980s. As a result of these familial and political connections, there is more information available concerning O'Brien than is the case with many of the others in this grouping.

Gerald O'Brien was born in West Ham, London, in 1910.[9] His father Ted was a successful stonemason, and the family moved to Cornwall Gardens, Kensington, in the late 1920s. In his autobiography, Garrett FitzGerald recalled visiting his London relations as a child in the 1930s, when his aunt Ciss, Gerald's mother, took in paying guests from the continent on the top floor of their Kensington home, lending 'a cosmopolitan air to this spacious house, the large first floor balcony of which was a family gathering-place on summer evenings'.[10] The O'Briens prospered sufficiently to endow Gerald with a private income of £300 per annum when he reached the age of majority.

Gerald was widely regarded as a brilliant young man and one who was possessed of great charm.[11] At the age of 21, he qualified as a chartered accountant and within two years was running his own practice based in Denman Street, W1, close to Piccadilly Circus. This placed him in Soho, the primary leisure district of London criminal underworld. O'Brien's charisma assisted him in both his licit and illicit enterprises and was an essential ingredient for the successful nightclub host. By the early 1930s, he had apparently grown bored with the staid world of accounting, and in 1932 was involved in his first marginal enterprise, a bottle party at Burlington Gardens in Mayfair.[12] This was followed shortly afterwards by a similar venture based in a New Bond Street flat.[13] The subsequent year saw him advertising in *The Times* for £600 with which to start up a new venture.[14] In 1935, in a precarious attempt to raise funds, O'Brien narrowly escaped a conviction for fraud. Together with three conspirators from the nightclub world, he obtained jewellery worth over £1500 by cheque. The four then pawned the jewellery and used the £700 cash raised to set up a club. In court, O'Brien explained that he was awaiting a large

[9] Biographical details such as date of birth were obtained from www.ancestry.co.uk, accessed 06.06.2015.

[10] G. FitzGerald, *Just Garret* (Dublin: Liberties Press, 2011), p. 19.

[11] *Daily Express* 8 July 1937, p. 9.

[12] *Times* 20 April 1932, p. 11. The bottle party was a 1930s invention that largely replaced the nightclub, finding a way to circumvent the licencing laws. See p. 123, *passim*.

[13] *Daily Mirror* 6 August 1932, p. 7.

[14] *Times* 17 March 1933, p. 1.

sum which he was owed and would have paid off the jeweller as soon as funds arrived; in the meantime, however, he had been very short of cash.[15] In the event, all four defendants were acquitted.[16]

In the early 1930s, O'Brien was one of the instigators (arguably the principal instigator) of the bottle party scheme for evading London's strict alcohol and entertainment licencing laws, which were perceived as oppressive by many of those drawn to the capital's nightlife.[17,18] Henceforth, Gerry, as he was widely known, turned his accounting and legal skills toward identifying and exploiting loopholes in the regulatory architecture governing London's nightlife and to providing consumer services at its margins. According to an acquaintance at the *Daily Express*, O'Brien was at this juncture living in a suite at the elite Grosvenor House Hotel; he owned a Rolls-Royce and earned around ten thousand pounds per annum.[19] The West End life involved Gerry O'Brien not only in the supply of marginal alcohol and entertainment services but of illegal drugs, to which he became addicted, and for the possession and 'wilful concealing' of which he was prosecuted in 1937.[20] At C Division's Vine Street station, where the Clubs Branch was based, Superintendent Dalton noted that, 'Gerald O'Brien is a well-known character in the club world, and any venture of his is almost bound to be on the wrong side of the law.'[21]

It was in the West End club world that O'Brien met dance hostess Bella Gold (1911–n/k). Bella's parents were Russian Jews who had emigrated to the UK in the early twentieth century; the 1911 census records them living at Stepney, where her father Solomon worked in the 'cap making trade'. Bella has left behind her little in the way of historical

[15] *Times* 13 March 1935, p. 8.

[16] *Hull Daily Mail* 26 March 1935, p. 12.

[17] H. B. Spear, *Heroin Addiction Care and Control* quotes Frank Thornton, one of Spear's colleagues at the Drugs Inspectorate, to the effect that O'Brien was the originator of the bottle party system, p. 52.; Fabian, *London After Dark* gives Eustace Hoey, another well-known West End nightclub entrepreneur, as the instigator, p. 17. There are various other claimants, too—it is likely, in fact, that there was no single originator behind the bottle party but rather several operators in the West End night-time economy who studied the licencing laws and identified a similar legal loophole.

[18] TNA MEPO 2/4487, 'Illegal sales of liquor at West End night bar: imprisonment for defendant already serving sentence for drug offences'. The bottle party system is described below.

[19] *Daily Express* 8 Jul 1937, p. 9.

[20] TNA MEPO 3/1056, Metropolitan Police telegram, 7 July 1937.

[21] TNA MEPO 2/4487, Memorandum, Vine Street 5 March 1937.

records; as Marek Kohn remarked of the subjects of *Dope Girls*, many of these drug users 'were just the sort of people who leave nothing after them, not even descendants'.[22] Like O'Brien, Bella was drawn to the West End, where she was living by the early 1930s and where she picked up five convictions for soliciting between 1931 and 1936.[23] The following year found her working in West End nightclubs and living in Connaught Mews, part of the up-market Connaught Village near Marble Arch; the address reflected Bella's improved financial circumstances and coincided with her alleged involvement in the supply of drugs. She was arrested in October 1937 when the Mews flat was raided by Detective Sergeant Arthur 'Len' Dyke of Scotland Yard and drugs including heroin, cocaine and Indian hemp were found. After the court case, she dropped from view.[24]

The last of the well-known figures in the network was Constance Freda Roberts (1911–1967), though her primary involvements seem to have been as friend and lover to the main protagonists and consumer of drugs.[25] Freda (she did not use her first name) had been born in the Yorkshire town of Bridlington; her father was a master mariner, killed in the First World War when his ship was torpedoed.[26] At the age of 17, she eloped with a bit-part actor and fled south to London, drawn to the lights and the opportunity of a less mundane life. Like so many others, she gravitated to the West End and was employed as a dance hostess at Romano's nightclub on the Strand and later at the Bag O'Nails club in Soho, both famous venues.[27] According to Spear, 'Len' Dyke (now working at the Drugs Branch) called her 'The toast of the West End', the implication being that she was a 'good time girl'.[28] Working in nightclubs and immersed in the West End life, she met the popular singer Al Bowlly at a party.[29] Following a 'whirlwind romance', they were married at St Martin's Registry Office, London, in December 1931. The marriage did not last long, Freda having allegedly been discovered by Bowlly

[22] M. Kohn, *Dope Girls*, p. 7.

[23] *Times* 11 October 1937, p. 9.

[24] *Daily Mail* 11 October 1937, p. 8; *Daily Express* 14 October 1937, 1.; *Daily Express* 18 October 1937, p. 5.

[25] H. B. Spear, *Heroin Addiction Care and Control*, p. 52.

[26] *Daily Express* 13 October 1938, p. 13; *Times* 13 October 1938, p. 4.

[27] C. Breese, *Hutch* (London: Bloomsbury, 1999) p. 83.

[28] H. B. Spear, *Heroin addiction: Care and Control*, p. 52.

[29] *Daily Express* 28 November 1951, p. 3.

in flagrante delicto on the wedding night.[30] It was her brief relationship with Bowlly that resulted in her appearance in a few of the memoirs from this period and prompted the press to run didactic stories of her drug career and spectacular downfall.

Based on the information provided to him by his older colleagues who recalled the 1930s West End drug scene, Spear estimated the numbers involved in this network to be no more than 20–25, many working in nightclubs.[31] Most of the participants consumed their opiates by means of insufflation or sniffing and preferred heroin to the morphine favoured in the Chelsea sets. They also used cocaine and Indian hemp, and their consumption was essentially social, taking place in what the press termed 'snuff parties'.[32] In addition, sniffing could be carried out swiftly and discretely at a club, and left no tell-tale marks on the body to be identified by police and medical examinations. This network avoided the kind of public drug use that their bohemian cousins sometimes practised, though they were equally remote from the respectable medical addiction with which the 1930s have often been associated by academic researchers.

It is unclear how long the network lasted: it seems likely that the supply function, which was at the heart of it, ended when both O'Brien and Gold were prosecuted in 1937. Each claimed that they had been using drugs for about four months, which would make it a very short-lived operation. However, this stretches credulity; putting together a network of 20–25 people took time. Moreover, O'Brien's continual financial difficulties, which had been on and off for some years, tend to point in the direction of a considerable drug habit. Unlike the drugs prescribed by doctors and dispensed through pharmacists, the price and purity of illicit drugs varied, placing more of a strain on personal finances. It is interesting that the group chose to source their drugs illegally despite this—a decision that was probably made both in order to avoid the police monitoring implicit in the licit system and because of the risky pleasures taken in pursuit of the illicit, a form of stimulation toward which it seems clear that O'Brien and probably Gold were drawn.

[30] *Cocktails with Elvira: Elvira Barney and her circle* https://elvirabarney.wordpress.com/2012/01/12/freda-roberts/.

[31] H. B. Spear, *Heroin Addiction: Care and Control* p. 52.

[32] Indian hemp was the name for cannabis.

Functioning of the West End Network

How then did the network operate, and what were the roles of these individuals? Firstly, the group's core business was, like that of its Chelsea counterpart, the consumption of drugs. However, unlike the Chelsea group, the West End network did not rely upon script doctors to obtain its drugs but rather sourced their supplies illicitly. The network was, therefore, as concerned with supply as it was with use. Both Gerry O'Brien and Bella Gold had visited Paris and had contacts in the illicit drug trade based there. During their excursions, they had encountered two American expatriates, Louis Carpenter and Johnny Fussell, who were drug traffickers living in Montmartre.[33] Carpenter and Fussell were based at the Hotel Oria in the Rue Pigalle, Pigalle being a major entertainment area and the hub of the city's commercial sex trade.

On June 30, 1937, while returning to London on the boat train, O'Brien was detained by customs officials at Newhaven. He had been visiting his Paris suppliers and was found to be in unlawful possession of six grammes of heroin. Bail was strongly opposed by the police, and he was remanded in custody before appearing at Lewes Police court on July 7, 1937. West End detectives were summoned to the court at Lewes to give evidence as to O'Brien's character and criminal history, but despite a persuasive performance in the dock, he was sentenced to six months' imprisonment.[34]

These visits to Paris were regular and had been going on for some time, though precise details (such as dates) are unknown. In addition, Bella Gold frequently received stocks of heroin, cocaine and cannabis by letter from the same source. When her flat was raided in October 1937, police discovered packages containing drugs that had been sent from Paris. The combination of visits and packages kept the network supplied, though it is impossible to estimate the quantities coming into London by these means. The trade from Paris, either by the boat train or by letter, was the major route for illicit drug supplies in the 1930s. Tom Driberg, writing as *Daily Express* columnist 'William Hickey', reported his encounter with an anonymous individual who had been 'a heroin addict for some years' and who was sceptical of press reports regarding major London drug rings about to

[33] TNA MEPO 3/1038, Case number No.964- Seizures at Newhaven, UK, in July, October and December 1937.

[34] TNA MEPO 3/1056, Metropolitan Police Telegram 7 July 1937.

be 'cleaned up'. He told Driberg that there were no large-scale trafficking rings like those after the Great War; instead, 'it was simply a matter of ringing up a doctor' of which he knew some 20, or, 'I could telephone to a number in Paris, order the stuff, promising to send cash'.[35] Knowing as he did many of the bright young people, Driberg's information was probably reliable. In addition, documentary evidence remains of other known cases of French suppliers who serviced London addicts by mailing letters containing heroin and cocaine; in July 1937 two traffickers, Henri Taddeo and Marcel P., were each sentenced to four months' imprisonment when found with a hundred grammes of heroin and the same quantity of cocaine in packages destined for the UK.[36]

In addition to his heroin retailing, O'Brien was a proprietor of bottle parties, a type of nightlife entertainment that was prevalent in the 1930s and at which drugs were allegedly made available to customers. According to Detective Sergeant Dyke, drugs were also retailed from Gold's flat in Connaught Mews. These arrangements were neatly symmetrical: supplies were bought in Paris and sold in or through London at night-time venues, some of them controlled by the network. Most of Spear's estimated 20–25 participants would have been retail customers of these drugs, many involved in the night-time economy. However, the bulk of the profits extracted from this system probably went on taking care of the principals' own drug habits.

As will be clear from the foregoing, this network was immersed in the clubs and parties of Soho and Mayfair. It is necessary to examine this zone more closely in order to understand the emergence of the group, its operations and its relationships with the regulatory authorities.

The West End Life

According to the post office, the West End of London is identical to the postal district of W1, being made up of Mayfair, Marylebone and Soho, and includes the shop-lined thoroughfares of Oxford Street, Regent Street, Tottenham Court Road and other famous names. However, the district has been mapped differently according to varying institutional, social and cultural imperatives. As cultural geographer Bronwen Edwards has

[35] *Daily Express* 9 September 1938, 'William Hickey column', p. 6.

[36] TNA MEPO 3/1038, 'League of Nations Advisory Committee on traffic in opium and other dangerous drugs: quarterly summaries from April1 to June 30th 1937' Case no. 674.

observed, 'The West End existed most coherently and meaningfully not as a precise territory, but as an imagined or represented place. It was the area of London associated with entertainment, shopping and fashionable living.'[37] However, alongside this consumer culture, another, darker form of consumption existed in the alleys, courtyards and basement clubs of Soho and increasingly, as the 1930s drew on, in the flats of Mayfair. This shadowy dimension of consumption included a variegated menu of sexual services, as well as unlicenced alcohol, gambling and drugs. As Inspector Robert Fabian of Scotland Yard stated: 'The Square Mile of Vice, we call it – Soho and the West End – where you can buy anything and see everything....'[38] The visibility of this economy was heightened at night, when the zone was transfigured by shimmering advertising displays, the syncopated rhythms of jazz music, smoky cellar clubs and the possibility of transgressive encounters in which hedonistic tastes and proclivities were given full scope. This was acutely so when experience was intensified and mediated by the action of drugs such as cannabis, heroin and cocaine, which became, for some, an adjunct to the excitement of the metropolitan night.

For certain individuals and groups, like O'Brien, Gold and their associates, the West End provided the context for a specialised existence, where a living could be had without resorting to conventional work with its routines and timetables, its hierarchies and tedium. This was an insecure, precarious living organised around the supply of illicit or borderline services, but it was flexible, possessed an outlaw glamour and offered an individualised freedom that could only be enjoyed within the circumscribed space of the square mile of pleasure, far from the respectability and domesticity of the expanding suburbs. The West End life was regarded by both participants and the authorities of law and medicine as something other than a regular mode of life. Drugs were not a necessary part of the West End life, but they were usually present and available, and were, it seems, tolerated as another ingredient in the carnival of vice that the district housed.

When West End addicts faced prosecution, they felt compelled to make promises to the courts to quit their mode of life and return to a

[37] B. Edwards, *Making the West End Modern: Space, Architecture and Shopping in 1930s London*. (Unpublished PhD Thesis, London: University of the Arts, 2004), p. 35.

[38] R. Fabian, *London After Dark: An intimate record of night life in London, and a selection of crime stories from the casebook of Ex-Superintendent Robert Fabian* (Kingswood, Surrey: Naldrett 1954), p. 10.

respectable and 'normal' existence. Bella Gold informed the magistrate, the same Morgan Griffith Jones who had in 1932 sent Brenda Dean Paul to prison, that she was 'through with the night club game' and that her family was going to help her to 'be happy in a normal regular life'.[39]

At the Margins of the Night-Time Economy: Bottle Parties

The bottle parties organised by O'Brien had their origins in the nightclubs of the jazz age. Historian Judith Walkowitz argues that just prior to the First World War, a small group of licit bohemian nightclubs appeared amongst the restaurants and cafes of the West End. With the outbreak of war, the DORA licencing regulations pushed drinking and dancing underground, both literally and figuratively. Unregistered clubs mushroomed in their hundreds in Soho and adjacent areas; occupying attics and basements, they 'prided themselves on their un-English atmosphere'.[40] Continuing in the early interwar years, these spaces became an integral part of London's entertainment industry; as Walkowitz comments, nightclubs, particularly those of Kate Meyrick, were 'icons of twenties nightlife'.[41]

Walkowitz takes issue with those such as contemporary commentator Patrick Balfour, who contended that the demise of the Meyrick clubs at the close of the 1920s represented the end of London's interwar nightlife.[42] On the contrary, by the mid-1930s, the worst of the economic depression was over; London's nightlife enjoyed something of a golden age during these years.[43] Paris was slow to recover from economic austerity, while Berlin, which had been the epicentre of the 1920s hedonistic culture, fell under the austere grip of National Socialism.

Despite this flowering of London's nightlife, the struggle between a pleasure-driven consumer culture and the imperatives of metropolitan security went on.[44] The nightclubs of the 1920s had experienced continuous

[39] *Daily Express* 18 October 1937, p. 5.

[40] J. R. Walkowitz, *Nights Out: Life in Cosmopolitan London* (New Haven & London: Yale University Press, 2012), p. 214.

[41] Walkowitz, *Nights Out*, p. 214.

[42] P. Balfour, *Society Racket: A critical survey of modern social life* (London: Long 1933) *passim*.

[43] A. Jenkins, *The Thirties* (London: Heinemann, 1976), p. 149.

[44] J. Schlor, *Nights in the Big City: Paris, Berlin, London 1840–1930* (New York: Reaktion, 1998).

pressure from the authorities, particularly under the regime of Home Secretary William Joynson-Hicks.[45] The regulation of alcohol consumption was restrictive, with the controls imposed during the First World War remaining in place except for minor relaxations flowing from the 1921 Act, which allowed London pubs to open until 11.00 pm or until 12.30 am if food was served with drinks. In response to this repressive regulatory apparatus, a new type of night-time venue that sought to evade the constraints of alcohol licencing (and the restrictions on music and dancing) began to appear in the early 1930s. It was known as the bottle party.[46]

The licencing regulations of the period were tight but did not cover private parties—a fact exploited with enthusiasm by the originators of the bottle party system, who circumvented the law to make alcohol, dancing and music available throughout the night, and were able to turn an often very handsome profit in the process. The bottle party system varied but involved the following: the venue was a private premises; it was not registered as a club or licenced to sell alcohol by the local magistrates. A few days prior to the planned event, invitations were sent out to guests, along with an order form requesting party-goers to authorise the organisers to purchase alcohol for them in advance; the wines, spirits and liqueurs would then be made available to them at the party, where they would pay the organisers for this service—sometimes at up to twice the original price. However, there was a tendency to dispense with the formal requirements of the system, which had kept it just about legal. As time passed, these requirements became a facade; as Richard Davenport-Hines puts it, 'Customers pretended to be there by prior invitation and drank alcohol which they had supposedly ordered earlier.'[47] In fact, guests were simply allowed in on the door, purchasing drinks from the organisers who had laid in a stock for that purpose. This violated the terms of the private party, as did the live music and dancing that was often laid on throughout the night.[48]

[45] J. Gardiner, *The Thirties: An Intimate History of Britain* (London: Harper, 2010), p. 629.

[46] R. Graves & A. Hodge, *The Long Weekend: The Living Story of the Twenties and Thirties* (Harmondsworth: Penguin, 1970; first published in 1940), pp. 226–227.

[47] R. Davenport-Hines, *An English Affair: Sex, Class and Power in the Age of Profumo* (London: Harper Press 2013), p. 142.

[48] A key decision on the legality of bottle parties was arrived at by Frederick Mead in 1933, when the famous 'Old Florida' nightclub in South Bruton Street, Mayfair, closed down and reopened as a private premises. The venue was henceforth organised as a bottle party, and in

The central role in the development of the bottle party played by O'Brien was demonstrated by a 1932 court case, in principle confirming their legality, which involved O'Brien and his associate, upper-class dance hostess Gwendoline Burke-Mills. On August 5, the two appeared at Marlborough Street in relation to a bottle party held at Burke-Mills' apartment in New Bond Street, Mayfair. She was charged with supplying alcohol without a licence, and he with aiding and abetting. The magistrate was Frederick Mead, that self-proclaimed defender of Victorian morality, in the year before his retirement. 'A number of fashionably dressed people occupied seats in court', observed the *Daily Mirror*.[49] The bottle party was indeed a fashionable institution, and as in the Dean Paul drug cases, the court appearance was at the centre of an intense cultural conflict over the regulation of consumption of intoxicants for pleasure; it received widespread press coverage.[50]

The entire prosecution of Burke-Mills and O'Brien was controversial. Once again Driberg weighed into the debate in his *Daily Express* society column. He was highly critical of the case, writing: 'Laymen visiting police courts must always be surprised by the immense amount of time spent in administering laws which are not concerned in any way with crime – as an ordinary man of the world would interpret the word.' He included the bottle party in this category. 'Meanwhile', he added, 'crime increases'.[51]

Drugs and the Nightlife

Drugs had been associated with the London nightclub scene since the First World War. Marek Kohn has explored this association, which has also been taken up recently by Lucy Bland, and may be further demonstrated by reference to both popular newspaper representation and expert medical discourse produced at the time.[52] In the wake of Freda Kempton's 1922 death from cocaine overdose, the *Daily Express* had warned its readers of 'Dancing, Dope and Death' in London's nightclubs, with their 'blasted lives of girls', while in 1930 the same newspaper carried stories of those

a test case, magistrate Frederick Mead found the system legal if carried out strictly according to these arrangements. *Gloucester Citizen* 28 July 1933, p. 10.

[49] *Daily Mirror* 6 August 1932, p. 7.

[50] *Times* 17 September 1932, p. 17; *Daily Mirror* 17 September 1932, p. 5; Daily *Mirror* 15 August 1932, p. 4; *Times* 15 August 1932, p. 7.

[51] *Daily Express* 6 August 1932, p. 13.

[52] M. Kohn, *Dope Girls, passim.*

'Driven Mad by Hashish' as a result of their attendance at 'Drug Orgies in London's Underworld'.[53,54] Meanwhile, from an expert medical perspective, Dr Nathan Raw, speaking at the May 1931 meeting of the Medico-Legal Society presided over by the Home Office addiction consultant Sir William Willcox, celebrated the fact that West End nightclubs used by addicts and pedlars were supposedly being swept away by the 'Byng broom'.[55] This was reference to the crusade of puritanical Home Secretary William Joynson-Hicks and his ally, Metropolitan Police Commissioner Lord Byng; the clubs responded by temporarily relocating to the suburbs and resorts along the Thames, such as Maidenhead.[56]

Rather than a simple matter of proximity, however, the relationship of nightclubs and drugs was mediated by their position in the marginal zone of the night-time economy. The illicit nature of the alcohol supply in this context, and the edgy conviviality it lubricated, fed into the tolerance and normalisation of other illegalities. The aura of revolt surrounding unlicenced alcohol linked it with the heroin, cocaine and hashish which were then circulating in the West End, binding them together as objects of unlawful consumption. This linkage was strengthened by the fact that each of these substances was in practice almost entirely unregulated at a time well within living memory—just prior to the First World War, when pub opening hours were principally a matter for the judgement of the individual landlord and opiates and cocaine could readily be purchased from pharmacies.[57] With the advent of alcohol prohibition in the USA and an unpopular regulatory system imposed on drinking in the UK, alcohol drew closer once again to the forbidden drugs and joined them in their illicit glamour.

Bottle parties provided subcultural spaces where behaviours that were not tolerated in the mainstream society were permitted, encouraged, explored. These included unlicenced all-night drinking; promiscuous sexual adventure; social mixing across class, gender and ethnic boundaries; the buying, selling and use of dangerous drugs; erotically charged dancing; and so on. These parties were regarded as centres of vice and deviance

[53] *Daily Express* 11 March 1922, p. 1.

[54] *Daily Express* 6 November 1930, p. 8.

[55] 'Medico-Legal Society' *Lancet* 217, 5623 (1931), pp. 1241–1243.

[56] M. Sweet, *Shepperton Babylon: The Lost Worlds of British Cinema* (London: Faber and Faber, 2006) pp. 47–52.

[57] J. Nicholls, *The Politics of Alcohol: A history of the drink question in England* (Manchester: Manchester University Press, 2009) pp. 150–160, 180, *passim*.

from which social and cultural disorder threatened to spread out and infect the wider metropolis, posing a series of problems for governance that centred around the risks inherent in the modern urban environment, with sexual and intoxicatory practices and identities developing.

Although bottle parties spread to provincial towns and cities, they remained concentrated in the West End, and the cultural icon of the bottle party was understood as a London phenomenon that had replaced the nightclubs of the 1920s as an emblematic figure of the new decade and of the modern metropolis.

Dance Hostesses

So, in the 1930s, bottle parties proliferated across the West End, taking over the entertainment and symbolic functions of the 1920s nightclub. A vital ingredient in these environments was the presence of the dance hostess.[58]

Employed by the bottle party organisers, the hostesses danced with clients, in addition to 'sitting out', that is, accompanying male guests at their tables by engaging in drinking and conversation and assuming the status of a glamorous companion. They were paid a moderate basic wage but could earn considerable sums over and above this by means of tips and commission. They encouraged clients to purchase champagne and cocktails, kept the waiters busy and generally lubricated the party machinery. In addition, gifts such as chocolates were made available by the club to which the guests could treat the hostesses, a percentage going to the girl herself. All of this consuming and spending was stimulated by the erotic allure of the dance hostesses, and perhaps their most important function was to imbue the environment with sexual promise and potential. The more that was consumed, the more the hostesses earned.

They were highly ambivalent cultural figures. Writer and feminist social commentator Ethel Mannin wrote a novel centred on the life of a dance hostess, in which the figure was popularly characterised as 'the next best thing to a prostitute'.[59] Meanwhile, in a 1931 case, Justice McCardle

[58] For early accounts of the dance hostess role at the Meyrick clubs of the 1920s, see K. Meyrick, Secrets *of the 43 Club* (Dublin: Parkgate, 1994, first published 1933), pp. 146–155; and R. Carlish, with A. Bestic, *King of Clubs* (London: Elek Books, 1962), p. 36, *passim*. Carlish was Kate Meyrick's manager at the 43 club and gives a less rosy account of the role of the dance hostesses than her own.

[59] E. Mannin, *Julie: The Story of a Dance Hostess* (London: Hutchinson, 1940) p. 69.

typified the views of the judiciary in branding the dance hostess system a 'disgrace to the city of London' and 'a direct incitement to young girls to go beyond the bounds of restraint'.[60] However, the availability of dance hostesses for commercial sex varied greatly, as did their class and social status, which stretched from the daughters of the rentier class to street prostitutes, depending on the type of party and its clientele.

The Met's raid on the New Bond Street bottle party in 1932 attracted a great deal of press attention, owing in part to the Mayfair location and the smart set involved and in part because the detectives visited the party in plain clothes.[61] The press reporting of events at the party illustrates something of the hostess role in practice. When the male police officer, the aptly named PC Cavalier, sat down at a table, Gwendoline Burke-Mills brought over a dance hostess and introduced her. She sat with the policeman and he began to order lager, but the hostess intervened: 'Shall we have some brandy?' Shortly afterwards the police raiding squad entered the room; the hostess told clients, 'It is a raid. Don't give your right names and addresses.'[62] It is apparent that the hostesses could be useful in managing the clients in the event of police intervention, as well as in their more traditional decorative and suggestive functions.

Bottle Parties and the Retailing of Drugs

On the surface, bottle parties would have been ideal spaces in which to offer drugs for retail sale, and newspapers regularly provided such narratives of supply. It was alleged, said *The Times*, that 'cocaine and heroin are being sold at certain night clubs and dance halls'; since the war, claimed *The Times*, drug laws had been introduced that successfully stamped out the 'evil'. 'Lately, however', it warned its readers, 'there has been a revival of the trade…'.[63] Other accounts stressed the risks to the hostesses rather

[60] *Daily Mirror* 20 November 1931, p. 2.

[61] The newspapers were both intrigued by the undercover detectives, PC Cavalier and Woman Patrol Dean, who were on surveillance duty at the venue, and outraged by the officers passing themselves off as upper class and quaffing champagne (on one night they allegedly consumed four bottles), and eating sandwiches at two shillings and sixpence each. *Daily Mirror* 15 August 1932, p. 4. For a discussion of the undercover policing of the 1920s Meyrick nightclubs, see H. Shore, '"Constable dances with instructress": the police and the Queen of Nightclubs in inter-war London', Social *History* 38,2 (2013) pp. 183–202.

[62] *Straits Times* 12 September 1932, p. 6.

[63] *Times* 28 June 1932, p. 11.

than the clientele: 'Most of the bottle parties are held in small stuffy rooms which become unduly crowded, and a girl who has spent the night dancing and drinking with her patrons finds that, about 3 or 4 in the morning she is feeling literally worn out.' This, we are told, is when the drug dealer pounces; interestingly, the drug in question in this latter report is not cocaine, which we might expect in this context, but Indian hemp, a cigarette 'with a kick in it'.[64] There were, in fact, indications of an increase in the availability of Indian hemp in the nightclub scene of the West End at the close of the 1930s. However, it is impossible to estimate its prevalence.[65]

Not everybody believed that drugs were available on the club and bottle party circuit. Dr Richard Starkie, the former police surgeon, abortionist and script doctor whom we encountered in Chap. 2, contributed an article to the *Daily Express* following his release from prison in 1932. Under a headline claiming that 500 'drug agents' were making 'an excellent living' in London by selling 'dope', Starkie alleged that 'many more people than the authorities imagine are taking drugs in London'. Heroin and cocaine were entering the capital in large quantities, he reported, but they were not being sold in clubs. 'There is an idea that some of the night clubs in London are places where drugs can be bought', said Starkie. 'That is altogether wrong. You might meet the people who would put you in the way of securing drugs, but there is no actual traffic at the clubs. The passing over is done at most respectable restaurants, at shops and railway stations.'[66]

While Starkie is not generally the most reliable of witnesses, on the nightclubs' point, his argument is plausible. The more or less open trading of drugs in nightclubs, mirroring the practices of the street drug market, was a popular theme whose practice was in reality confined to the most brazen of the 'wide' clubs, such as those described by criminal-turned-sociologist and journalist Mark Benney.[67] We know that bottle parties and nightclubs were raided regularly by the Met and that most police drug interventions derived from the use of informants.[68] In a geographically

[64] *Perth Sunday Times* 23 January 1938, p. 5.

[65] Mills, *Cannabis Nation*, p. 13.

[66] *Daily Express* 15 May 1930, p. 11.

[67] M. Benney, *Low Company: Describing the evolution of a burglar* (Horsham: Caliban, 1981; first published 1936) pp. 184–216.

[68] See Chap. 5 for a discussion of the use of informants.

limited area in which the numbers involved in the subculture were relatively tiny, discretion would have been essential in keeping a drug business afloat.

At the O'Brien bottle parties, while definitive evidence remains elusive, it is likely that something closer to the pattern of retail relationships described by Dr Starkie was employed. Both Gerry and Bella probably handled retail supplies; those closest to the centre of the network, who were regularly accessing the selection of drugs obtained from the Paris connection and retailed in London, would most likely have been able to pick up supplies directly at the clubs if they needed to. So, it is likely that some retail supply was carried on in these and similar venues. Generally, however, it is probable that arrangements were made for them to either visit the flat in Connaught Mews or to meet at some agreed place to collect these products.

Narrative and Counter-Narrative: Bella Gold in Court

Detective Sergeant Dyke, the Met's leading expert in drugs at this juncture, who was to join the Home Office Drugs Branch early in the Second World War, made sure that the seriousness of the Bella Gold case was evident in his testimony when the case came up in October 1937. He testified that Gold's associates were drug addicts, that she was looked upon by the police not as an addict but 'quite definitely' as a trafficker and that the Met suspected strongly that drugs were sold from her apartment. The Home Office, in addition, were said to take a very serious view of the case.[69]

Dyke reminded the court of Bella's repeated soliciting offences between 1931 and 1936, and reported that he had found 26 airmail letters from Paris in the flat, 11 of which contained 'veiled references' to the sending of drugs. These veiled references were significant; the letters utilised drug argot, with mentions of 'jive', 'blowing the top off', 'getting high' and so on.[70] This was the vocabulary of the US drug scene, and its use shows that, along with jazz music and dance, it had penetrated the discourse of the vicious addicts of Paris and London. This is contrary to the analysis of contemporaries such as the Chicago sociologist Alfred Lindesmith, who

[69] *Times* 18 October 1937, p. 9.
[70] *News of the World* 10 October 1937, p. 2.

contended that there was no drug subculture in the UK and therefore no drug argot.[71] Dyke also sought to establish Gold's connection with Gerry O'Brien, who had featured repeatedly in court and in newspapers since the previous July; it was a linkage that would do her case no good, since O'Brien was represented as both a major heroin trafficker and the mastermind behind the bottle party system.

Nonetheless, the defence established a counter-narrative that turned out to be successful. Bella had become ill through working in the dusty club environment, with its late hours and cigarette smoking. She had developed a bronchial problem and, while in Paris, had met 'one of those pernicious beasts who live by selling these drugs'.[72] A sniff of white powder had instantaneously relieved her discomfort, and she had made an arrangement with the 'beast' in question to mail her regular quantities. As the *Daily Mail* reported, 'Soon she was in their clutches.'[73]

This is the classic alibi, used in countless drug cases in the interwar period. A girl (usually) is given opiates (generally in Paris) to manage or cure an illness, becoming thereby a victim addict (as opposed to a vicious addict), and ultimately finding herself in court. Although the typical narrative involves the intervention of a French doctor, in this instance even the 'pernicious' trafficker assumes what is in effect a therapeutic role, albeit a misguided one. The magistrate, Mr Morgan Griffith Jones, who had been so unmoved by the plight of Brenda Dean Paul, was in this case softened by the 'titian haired' Miss Gold and was persuaded to sentence her to two years' probation.[74] Her case was no doubt assisted by her ardent and reiterated rejection of the West End life: 'I am through with the night club game', she told the magistrate, 'I shall never have anything more to do with drugs. I've learned my lesson.'[75,76]

[71] A. R. Lindesmith, 'The Argot of the Underworld Drug Addict' *Journal of Criminal Law and Criminology*, 29,2, (1938) pp. 261–278.

[72] *Daily Mail* 11 October 1937, p. 9.

[73] *Daily Mail* 18 October 1937, p. 9.

[74] *Daily Express* 14 October 1937, p. 1. The evidence in this case was, incidentally, lacking in coherence. The Paris trafficker allegedly gave Bella Gold a 'white powder' which alleviated her bronchial cough; this was almost certainly heroin, which was known to be an effective therapeutic for such ailments. The trafficker then arranges for her to receive regular supplies of Indian hemp by post—which is *not* an effective remedy in such ailments. It is clear that the narrative is flawed, but whether this is at the level of the court or the newspapers is impossible now to say.

[75] *Daily Express* 18 October 1937, p. 5.

[76] *Daily Mail* 18 October 1937, p. 9.

Subcultural Geography of Drugs in the Late 1930s: Soho and Mayfair

Artist, model and writer Nina Hamnett, who had taken drugs with Aleister Crowley's network in the 1920s, was allegedly asked by two bohemian sightseers in Fitzrovia where they might see some 'dope fiends'.[77] 'I think you had better go back to Mayfair if you want to find people who take drugs', she replied.[78] There may have been some humour in her response. Nonetheless, by the 1930s it was certainly in Soho and Mayfair that the white drug trade was centred, in a zone stretching from the eastern end of Archer Street in Soho to Shepherd Market in Mayfair. Archer Street was where the musicians' union had its headquarters, and where an informal employment exchange functioned on the pavements of Archer Street itself; musicians would meet, talk and smoke in the street's cafes.[79] Despite denials from those critics who favoured and defended jazz music, there was always considerable drug use amongst the musicians and other entertainers who performed in the clubs, hotels and restaurants of the West End. Superintendent Fabian identified The Nest nightclub in Kingly Street as the place where cannabis was first smoked in London, a story that was probably apocryphal but probably contained more than a germ of truth.[80] Freda Roberts described smoking the drug outside the Bag O'Nails—also in Kingly Street—where she worked in the mid-1930s.[81]

It is notable too that there appears to have been, in the late 1930s, a specific cluster of drug retailing based in the clubs and bottle parties close to Regent Street, on the boundary of the two districts, centred primarily on Fouberts Place and Kingly Street. Fouberts Place was where Gerry O'Brien set up the last of his club ventures prior to his arrest and prosecution for unlawful possession of heroin in July 1937. After O'Brien and his associates were shut down, a bottle party named the Brown Bomber set up in Fouberts Place; some time afterwards, this too was closed by the police after a tip-off was received warning them that a letter containing heroin

[77] N. Hamnett, *The Laughing Torso: Reminiscences of Nina Hamnett* (New York: Ray Long, 1932) p. 178.

[78] V. Nicholson, Among *the Bohemians: Experiments in Living 1900–1939* (London: Penguin, 2002) p. 272.

[79] Musicians' Union: A social history; Archer Street, London. http://www.muhistory.com/?p=344 Accessed 28.06.2015.

[80] Fabian, London After Dark, p. 20.

[81] *Daily Express* 29 November 1951, p. 3.

had been sent to the club from Paris. Robert Clement, an addict who was a patient of Dr Quinlan, ran the venue in partnership with the black American entertainer Thomas Brookins.[82] The police followed up this anonymous call from Paris and seized the heroin. The two were sent to prison, later appealing their sentences on the ground that a London gangster named Jimmy Orr had arranged the whole thing, allegedly because he himself was using the club to supply heroin and Clement and Brookins had discovered this and banned him.[83] Whether or not this was true, there is no way to tell; the appeal was, however, successful. Either way, the point is that the club was clearly linked to the dealing of heroin, as was the area immediately surrounding it.

The Rise and Fall of 'Mayfair Man'

In the reporting of the O'Brien network's drug court appearances, the Mayfair location featured prominently and significantly. The cases played into a string of others that referenced the downward trend of the district; amongst the most important was the jewellery robbery involving four 'Mayfair playboys' from the smart set.[84] The four had robbed West End jeweller Etienne Bellenger by luring him to the Hyde Park Hotel on the pretext of a sale and then knocking him out, making their escape with some £13,000 worth of diamonds and other jewellery. Their public school educations, privileged lives and upper-class family backgrounds had been deployed by the press in making the crime appear especially heinous. Many of the press representations found its cause in their louche Mayfair lifestyle. It was a world of playboy gangsters, fast cocktail girls, nightclubs, gambling—all of it summarised in the figure of 'Mayfair Man'.[85]

There were many other cases and numerous representations invoking this figure: 'Good looking, twenty one year old…ex-public school boy, another victim of London's night life – expensive bottle parties, high-stakes gambling and glamorous but costly girlfriends.'[86] Questions were

[82] *Times* 16 March 1938, p. 9.

[83] *Daily Mail* 16 March 1938, p. 9.

[84] A. McLaren *Playboys & Mayfair Men: Crime, Class, Masculinity, and Fascism in 1930s London* (Baltimore, Johns Hopkins Press, 2017). This work was published after the writing of my own and covers the culture of 1930s Mayfair in greater depth.

[85] See, for example, *Times*, 16 February 1938, p. 18; *Daily Express* 19 February 1938, pp. 1, 3 & 5; *Daily Mirror* 19 February 1938, pp. 3, 6.

[86] *Daily Mirror*, 10 March 1938, p. 9.

asked in parliament alongside the alarm expressed in the press, with both calls for the use of corporal punishment and opposing arguments claiming that this sadistic practice would further erode what was best about British society.[87]

Alongside the rise of Mayfair Man and the drugs used in the locality, historian Stefan Slater notes an increasing movement of prostitution into Mayfair, with the police very active in their attempts to suppress the trade during this period. Vigorous attempts were made to 'clean up' Mayfair and Paddington in 1936, the year of the coronation, but these had been less than effective.[88] All of the anxieties articulated by the newspapers played into the problems associated with Mayfair and its amorality, and the degradation of the upper classes that it represented: these fed into the background of the reporting of Gerry O'Brien and his West End life, and textured the ways in which the case was understood.

The Night Bar and the End of the Network's Drug Business

O'Brien's last enterprise involved a club named the Night Bar and operated on a new variation of the bottle party scheme. Clients ordered two gallons of wine or spirits from a licenced wholesaler, which could legally stay open and serve all night and which was attached to the premises of the club. The customer then took delivery of one 96th part of it, equivalent to a large double, at a table in the club. The consumer was not required to pay for the remainder. This scheme had been tried out with some success at the Savile Hotel in Cork Street the previous October, and since then O'Brien and his associates had made extensive alterations to the premises in Fouberts Place, where the Night Bar opened in March 1937.[89] The Met sent detectives to investigate the venue on opening night, but they were unable to gain entry, ostensibly because they had no invitations but more likely because they were spotted as police officers.

[87] Hansard, *House of Commons Debate 3rd March 1938; Vol 332 ccl 274–5.*

[88] S. Slater, 'Pimps, Police and Filles de Joie: Foreign Prostitution in Interwar London' The *London Journal* 32,1 (2007), 53–74. pp. 63, 66, *passim.*

[89] *Times*, 7 December 1936, p. 11. The 'raid' was on the Savile Hotel's proprietress, who had left the hotel in the care of O'Brien only for him to turn it into a bottle party and 'disorderly house'. The report gives a first indication of threats from O'Brien, which suggest that there may have been a touch of gangsterism about his business practices.

When O'Brien became aware of police interest, he immediately disappeared to France, and it was on his return in July 1937 that he was apprehended by customs officials and arrested for possessing and wilfully concealing heroin. As noted above, this resulted in a six months' sentence of imprisonment. His defence was a variation on that deployed by Bella Gold and Brenda Dean Paul and involved difficulties in Paris; O'Brien claimed that he took heroin there because he had no money and was suffering from acute pangs of hunger. 'I had always had a horror of drugs', he stated in court, 'even though my friends all took them'.[90] Although the Lewes magistrates recognised Gerry O'Brien as 'brilliant, cultured and educated', they nonetheless imprisoned him. The Chairman of the magistrates declared that 'drug-taking is one of the most abominable practices any human being can conceive' and the public had to be protected.[91]

The Night Bar closed down in April 1937 and those involved were subject to a total of £568 in fines. O'Brien was brought to London in October by two warders from Lewes prison and appeared at Marlborough Street police court. He argued that the Night Bar was legal and that he had had no case to answer; Mr Boyd, the magistrate, did not agree, and he was sentenced to one month in prison, though this was to run concurrently to the heroin sentence he was currently serving.[92]

In that same October, Bella Gold was raided by Len Dyke, effectively ending the minor trafficking system operated by the West End network; Freda Roberts was prosecuted in the subsequent year. Roberts was found in possession of Indian hemp, although she confessed to being a heroin addict, and was sentenced to a £10 fine. As James Mills has observed, her defence in court closely resembled that of Bella Gold.[93] It was, indeed, well on the way to becoming a traditional formula for defence against drug charges in the 1930s and was often effective in keeping the defendant out of prison.

Freda Roberts' addiction would continue into the early 1960s. According to Spear, one of the addicts associated with the O'Brien network was still in receipt of prescriptions for morphine in 1994, though no details are given.[94] The others either found doctors to prescribe or had

[90] *News of the World*, 11 July 1937, p. 5.

[91] Ibid.

[92] *Morning Advertiser*, 23 October 1937, n.p.

[93] James H. Mills, *Cannabis Nation*, p. 21.

[94] H. B. Spear, *Heroin Addiction, Care and Control*, p. 52.

recourse to alternative illicit sources. The West End network was fragmented in the course of these vicissitudes, and ceased to exist as a unit, though isolated individuals reappeared in other groupings. The West End life continued to provide a fertile source for drug subcultural formation in the postwar years and retained its attraction for drug-centred lifestyles into the twenty-first century. Some of the criminal affiliates of O'Brien were to reappear in the 1940s when a number of attempts, albeit small, were made to transform the market deriving from script doctors into a larger-scale source of supply.

CHAPTER 5

The Regulation of Opiates Under the Classic British System, c.1920–c.1945

INTRODUCTION

The previous three chapters followed the emergence of script doctors and new white drug cultures in the 1930s. This chapter explores 'the other side of the coin', tracing the early history of a network of interlocking regulatory agencies and services that cooperated to try to curtail the activities of those groups and individuals supplying and using opiates for non-medical purposes. This web of powers included the Home Office Drugs Branch and the Metropolitan Police with its Chemist Inspection Officers and its specialist drug teams who were the predecessors of the drug squad formed after the Second World War.[1] These were supplemented by the Regional Medical Officers of the Ministry of Health who cooperated with the Drugs Branch to investigate cases of intensive or extended prescribing, usually identified by the Chemist Inspection Officers, the GMC and the ordinary generalist in what was then often private practice or a mixture of private and national health insurance or 'panel' patients.[2] It was a complex and dense network of forces that sought to regulate both drug consumers and the doctors whose prescribing formed their major source of supply.

[1] As previously discussed, the early opiate subculture was centred overwhelmingly on London, and it was the London-based regulators who were its main adversaries.

[2] The Pharmaceutical Society of Great Britain, then the professional body for pharmacists, was also involved in regulating chemists' shops from 1933, following the passage of the Pharmacy and Poisons Act. Its inspectors did not have authority over dangerous drugs, and so had little contact with script doctors or addicts. For this reason, they do not feature largely in this research.

C. Hallam, *White Drug Cultures and Regulation in London, 1916–1960*, https://doi.org/10.1007/978-3-319-94770-9_5

Not all drug users drew much regulatory attention; the compliant medical addict was largely left alone once the Home Office had researched the case and identified it as such. It was the 'vicious addicts', the formative subcultural groups, who rejected the constraints of the medical model that represented the major target. The regulatory agencies worked cooperatively, though there were often tensions between them over specific issues. As illustrated in the previous chapter, other forces also made significant informal contributions to the suppression of illicit drug use: various members of the public such as cab drivers, messenger boys, servants, hotel managers and so on, to which I have collectively referred as the lay culture of surveillance.

While many of the American commentators responsible for the construction of the concept of the 'British System' referred the term almost exclusively to the supply of opiates to addicts by doctors, the historical British System of drug control involved multiple structural elements, a point made previously by the psychiatrist Griffith Edwards.[3] The early decades of this network of juridical, medical and administrative controls have received relatively little historical attention with respect to their day-to-day operations and interactions. It is an imbalance I shall try to correct here. The actions of the 'vicious addicts'—those drug consumers of who were neither medical addicts suffering an iatrogenic illness nor healthcare professionals tempted by their proximity to powerful medications—and of the regulators who faced them can be properly understood only in relation to one another. Each time one side took a step in the dance that has now been played out for close to a century, the other responded with its own moves and counter-measures. On the control side, the Home Office was the responsible government department, and its Drugs Branch played a coordinating role in regulating the manufacture, supply and consumption of dangerous drugs within the classic British System. It also provided the necessary linkages with the international regulatory structure, which was at this time handled by the League of Nations.[4]

[3] G. Edwards, 'Some years on: evolutions in the "British System"', in D. J. West (ed) *Problems of drug abuse in Britain* (Cambridge: Cambridge University Press, 1978), pp. 1–2.

[4] W. B. McAllister, *Drug Diplomacy in the Twentieth Century: An international history* (London and New York: Routledge, 2000).

The Historiography of Interwar Opiate Regulation

The historiography of drug regulation in the UK is limited, at least until one reaches the postwar period. Moreover, components such as the role of police Chemist Inspection Officers and the Ministry of Health's Regional Medical Officers have been barely covered at all.

Henry 'Bing' Spear, who joined the Home Office Drugs Branch in 1952 and retired as its head in 1986, has so far written most extensively on the history of the organisation.[5] Spear possessed detailed knowledge of the workings of the Drugs Branch, derived from his own experience and his familiarity with some of the same archive sources utilised in the course of the present research. However, while he was a trenchant critic of the UK government's later policy direction in relation to drugs, Spear's analysis sits squarely within the institutional perspective of the Home Office in which he worked for 34 years, and shares uncritically many of its assumptions. While providing numerous 'clues' that were followed up with further research, Spear was, in the closing decades of the classical British System, a leading player, and his writings and interviews need to be understood in this context.

In her account of the Drugs Branch, Sarah Mars concentrates on the period since the 1960s, that is, the years following the demise of the classic British System.[6] Mars' narrative of its earlier stages is confined to a sketch, in keeping with the period on which her book is focused.[7] She points out that the Drugs Branch was 'the first arm of the British government to develop extensive expertise in drug misuse'.[8] She also notes, importantly, that although its staff did not possess medical qualifications, the Branch did develop 'its own internal expertise and views on appropriate prescribing'.[9] This included an implicit and informal set of opinions that helped to guide its judgement and conduct around the question of who was and who was not a script doctor. Mars also notes that the Branch

[5] H. B. Spear, *Heroin Addiction, Care and Control* and 'Conversation with Bing Spear: Journal Interview 20', *British Journal of Addiction* 83, (1988) pp. 473–482.

[6] S. G. Mars, *The Politics of Addiction: Medical Conflict and Drug Dependence in England since the 1960s* (Basingstoke: Palgrave Macmillan, 2012).

[7] Ibid., p. 90. Mars appears to claim that her focus on the later operations of the Drugs Branch results from a lack of archive materials; however, there are considerable archive resources dealing with the early years of the Branch available at the National Archives.

[8] Ibid., p. 98.

[9] Ibid., p. 104.

recognised that it was important to avoid being seen to be commenting on 'the well-defined turf of doctors' clinical judgment', and accordingly made use of existing medical views and evidence to represent its own positions.[10]

In his history of cannabis control and consumption in Britain, meanwhile, James Mills pays more attention to the origins and early workings of the Drugs Branch, finding its genesis in 'administrative wrangles in the wake of the 1920 legislation'.[11] Mills observes that the development of the Drugs Branch, even though its focus was chiefly on opiates and cocaine, established 'a well-developed state apparatus' that would be ready to respond when cannabis began to appear in Britain in larger quantities in the late 1940s. As we will see in the course of this research, the same cannot necessarily be said of the Drugs Branch a decade later when the second wave of opiate subculture took hold and proliferated. In this respect the Branch appears to have wilfully downplayed the growth of opiate addiction; even though it certainly knew that consumption was expanding, it neglected to place evidence of the fact before the Brain Committee during preparations for the Committee's first report.[12]

With regard to the police, the second of the main regulatory agencies, there is very little historical research that documents their dealings with drugs. The preeminent British police historian, Clive Emsley, has paid some attention to the policing of drug use in the interwar period, but has drawn largely on secondary sources in familiar cases, featuring, for example, the role of the press in constructing the mythic 'criminal mastermind'.[13] Police memoirs from the period regularly contain sections on drug trafficking and consumption but are highly stylised and structured by the narrative tropes of crime fiction.[14] While useful in certain ways—for example, in revealing police attitudes toward race and gender—they tell us little about the policing of drug users.

[10] Ibid., p. 105.

[11] J. H. Mills, *Cannabis Nation: Control and Consumption in Britain, 1928–2008* (Oxford: Oxford University Press 2012) p. 24.

[12] See Chap. 8 for discussion.

[13] C. Emsley, *Crime and Society in Twentieth-Century England* (Harlow: Pearson Education, 2011) pp. 119–20.

[14] See, for example, R. Fabian, *London After Dark: An intimate record of night life in London, and a selection of crime stories from the casebook of Ex-Superintendent Robert Fabian* (Kingswood, Surrey: Naldrett, 1954).

Much of the historical literature, framed by debates over the relative merits of a US 'penal' system as against a UK 'medical' one, focuses on the success or otherwise of the maintenance prescribing policy. Following the contours of Berridge's foundational analyses, it also stops at the Rolleston Report of 1926 and fails to engage with regulatory operations and changes between 1930 and the 1960s. More recent work, such as that of Sarah Mars, demonstrates a minimal engagement with the social and cultural elements that drew forth the drug control regime in the first place.

The Origins of the Home Office Drugs Branch

Press and state anxieties clustering around the use of cocaine by the British and allied armed forces in the capital had culminated in the passing of Defence of the Realm Act (DORA) regulation 40b, which restricted the possession of cocaine and opium to 'authorised persons'.[15] At the same time, a proclamation was issued forbidding the import of these drugs except under Home Office licence: the smuggling of opiates to the Far East on board British ships had also provided an incitement to government action.[16] These regulations required bureaucratic oversight and action, and this imperative initiated what would later become the Home Office Drugs Branch.

In the beginning, however, the system was established on a contingent basis; the government tried for over ten years to administer this work of oversight on the cheap, using ad hoc methods and temporary staff. The retirement of Sir Malcolm Delevingne, undersecretary of state at the Home Office with responsibility for drugs, along with that of the original inspector, Arthur Anderson, sent the branch into chaos in the early 1930s. Simultaneously, Britain's international obligations under the League of Nations treaties now required it to establish the Drugs Branch on a more secure basis. The Branch emerged from these transformations as a properly staffed and funded formal unit in the Home Office, with important domestic and international mandates.

The fact that the UK drug control regime had emerged in the context of the First World War and its aftermath had an important influence on the

[15] V. Berridge, 'War conditions and narcotics control: the passing of the Defence of the Realm Act regulation 40B' *Journal of Social Policy*, 7, (1978) pp. 285–304. M. Kohn, *Dope Girls*, pp. 34–44.

[16] V. Berridge, 'War conditions and narcotics control', pp. 293–5.

institutional culture of the Drugs Branch—an influence that was not always benign. The Branch tended, until the 1960s, to be backward looking and somewhat complacent, routinely locating the crisis of nonmedical drug use in the past, in the days before the dangerous drugs laws had been enacted and enforced. This was one of the factors that made it slow to react in the postwar period when changing circumstances required a different response.

Early Development of the Drugs Branch

In its early years, then, prior to the formal inception of the Drugs Branch in 1933, the administration of drug control was carried out under ad hoc arrangements and funded on a shoestring by a reluctant Treasury. In October 1916, a temporary administrative assistant named Arthur Anderson was employed by the Home Office to carry out duties under the provisions of DORA 40B and the proclamations controlling the import of opium and cocaine. He was joined in the following year by Frank Thornton, who became head of the Drugs Branch in 1943. Thornton had worked for Burgoyne Burbidges and Co. of East Ham, a wholesale druggist ('one of the largest in the country') that had close relations with the Home Office.[17] He was then employed by the Board of Trade, in the Chemical Section of the Import Restriction Department. These posts would equip him well for the work of the Drugs Branch.

In September of 1920, the Home Office and the Ministry of Health agreed that Anderson and Thornton should carry on the inspections required by the new Dangerous Drugs Act.[18] As noted by Mills, there was some dispute with the Treasury about the costs involved, the Treasury arguing that it was likely that the drug trade would be reduced to the point where the permanent employment of two inspectors would be unnecessary.[19] Nonetheless, with the support of Sir Malcolm Delevingne, the appointments went ahead, Anderson being employed as acting principal inspector and Thornton as his assistant. Two clerical support staff were also recruited. Delevingne, with his customary astringency, had reminded

[17] TNA HO 45/24948, Annual Report of the Home Office Drugs Branch for 1931.

[18] TNA HO 45/24761, passim. See also H. B. Spear *Heroin Addiction, Care and Control*, p. 35.

[19] J. H. Mills, (2012) *Cannabis Nation* p. 24. Such expectations illustrate the extraordinary faith that some of those working in the early drug control structures placed in the system's ability to effectively wipe out the nonmedical consumption of drugs.

the Treasury that the British government had entered into obligations under the International Opium Convention of 1912 to restrict the use of dangerous drugs to 'medical and legitimate' purposes, and required the administrative machinery to fulfil these obligations.[20] Delevingne's position was transmitted to the Treasury by one Mr Crapper at the Home Office: 'We (i.e. the British government) undertook to take certain steps to control the manufacture, sale, export and import of specified dangerous drugs and we are under an obligation to provide the necessary machinery for carrying out our commitments.'[21]

In 1926, Delevingne listed the following as the inspectors' duties: inspection of those manufacturing and wholesale chemists licenced under the 1920 Act and advice on the licencing of applicants, the issuing of export licences, the examination of the League of Nations statistical returns, miscellaneous work connected with administering the Act and the inspection of doctors' records in special cases. The police could be notified if it was judged appropriate, but generally it was believed that investigation of doctors by a fellow professional was preferable to a visit from the constabulary.[22] If the case required still further investigation, the Branch's inspectors would pursue it. So, from the earliest days of the Drugs Branch—prior to its official establishment in 1933—the unit worked in close collaboration with other state agencies, including the Ministry of Health and the police.

Although they had been authorised to examine pharmacy records under the Defence of the Realm legislation since 1917, it was in 1921 that the police were given responsibility to undertake the routine inspection of retail pharmacists' records of the dispensing of dangerous drugs. A circular was sent out by Delevingne informing chief constables of this new duty in August 1921. The decision was pragmatically driven: there were several thousand retail pharmacies to inspect, and the two civil servants then staffing the Branch could obviously not be expected to undertake all the work.[23] Instead, there was a new division of labour, with the police inspecting retail chemist shops and the Drugs Branch inspectors visiting licenced drug manufacturers and wholesalers. They also requested these licencees

[20] TNA HO 45/24761, Crapper to Gaitliff, 1 July 1921.

[21] Ibid.

[22] TNA HO 45/19983, DANGEROUS DRUGS AND POISONS: Dangerous Drugs Acts 1920 and 1923: application to doctors and dentists; inspection of records and stocks, 1921–1929.

[23] TNA HO 45/24948, Annual Report of Drugs Branch for 1930 Memo of 28.03.1930.

to notify them if they became aware of unusually large or extended provision of drugs to their own customers, particularly when those customers were retail chemists' shops, and the drugs were therefore likely to be going toward supporting addiction. Such reports were followed up by the Branch's inspectors and, in the case of doctors, by inspectors or RMOs.[24]

The job description supplied by Delevingne in 1926 was influenced by previous experience of administering the 1920 Act and by the provisions of the 1925 Opium Convention, which applied a regime of checking and certification to the import and export of narcotics within the extensive legal trade in these substances. These regulations were inscribed in domestic law by the Dangerous Drugs Act of 1925 (coming into force in 1928).

The Retirement of Delevingne and the Formal Creation of the Drugs Branch

The role of Delevingne in the establishment of the early drug control system is well known, and his importance can scarcely be exaggerated.[25] On the international scale, he was instrumental in the drafting and operation of the League of Nations system and the treaties that underpinned it; domestically, he oversaw everything that was related to these treaties in the UK.[26] Under Delevingne's direction, according to his contemporary Whitelegge of the Home Office, 'there was … set up, in effect, a separate expert compartment in which all knowledge and experience was concentrated'.[27]

In June 1932, with Delevingne's retirement fast approaching, high-level discussions were held at the Home Office concerning the future of the drug control arrangements. Aside from Sir Malcolm's departure, which was looming in less than six months, these discussions were

[24] TNA HO 45/24948, Annual Report of Drugs Branch for 1931.

[25] See W. B. McAllister, *Drug Diplomacy in the Twentieth Century: An international history* (London and New York: Routledge 2000); see also K. Bruun, L. Pan & I. Rexed, *The Gentlemen's Club: International Control of Drugs and Alcohol* (Chicago: University of Chicago Press, 1975) and P. Knepper, *International Crime in the 20th Century: The League of Nations Era*, 1919–1939 (Basingstoke: Palgrave Macmillan, 2011).

[26] The international system is often misunderstood as being a separate regime of drug control. In fact, the international conventions are not 'self-executing'; that is, in order to function, they require signatory states to enact national legislation. The two aspects of the system are therefore indissolubly interwoven.

[27] TNA HO 45/24761, Whitelegge to Harris, 14.07.1933.

provoked by a number of related developments that would impact upon the Branch's work: the retirement of the senior dangerous drugs inspector Arthur Anderson, which had just taken place, and the transfer to Private Secretarial work of Sir Austin Strutt, a Home Office legal advisor who was knowledgeable on drugs matters, were both significant. In addition, there was a new legislation to be dealt with: the Pharmacy and Poisons Act of 1933, which would generate considerable new work for the Home Office, and the UK's ratification of the 1931 Limitation Convention, requiring parties to establish a special administration to deal with drugs matters. Last but not least, the Home Office planned to 'divisionalise' or integrate the dangerous drugs staff into the broader civil service.

The most immediate legal demand on the government for establishment of the Drugs Branch on a firmer footing came from its ratification of the Convention for Limiting the Manufacture and Regulating the Distribution of Narcotic Drugs, 1931 (usually known as the 'Limitation Convention'). Article 15 of this treaty called upon its signatories thus:

> The High Contracting Parties shall, if they have not already done so, create a special administration for the purpose of:
>
> (a) Applying the provisions of the present Convention;
> (b) Regulating, supervising and controlling the trade in drugs;
> (c) Organising the campaign against drug addiction, by taking all useful steps to prevent its development and to suppress the illicit traffic.[28]

The Limitation Convention was intended to restrict the manufacture, imports and stocks of drugs to the country's medical needs. It would entail new and further duties for dangerous drugs staff, whom the UK had agreed to locate in a new, centralised administration.

When Delevingne announced his intention to retire, he also proposed a major structural reorganisation of the UK's drug control arrangements. This was to involve the 'divisionalisation' of the work—its integration into the mainstream of the civil service. The most important consequence of such a measure would be that staff working on dangerous drugs duties could be transferred to work elsewhere in the Home Office and into other departments. The planned reorganisation meant that there would be less

[28] *Convention for Limiting the Manufacture and Regulating the Distribution of Narcotic Drugs, Done at Geneva 9th July 1931. Entry into force 9th July 1933.*

funds coming from the Treasury, which was consequently in favour of the new scheme and promptly authorised it.

However, it quickly became clear that a reorganisation along these lines could not succeed. Those with experience of the drugs work believed that it was 'essentially different from the many other subjects which are dealt with administratively by the Home Office and that what we really need is a small group of experts'.[29] This was because the work was extremely complex and involved a great deal of international knowledge and contacts regarding both its licit and illicit aspects, and because the British representative at Geneva was also required to represent the colonies (apart from India, which was directly represented). It was evident that Delevingne had underestimated his own contribution to the smooth working of the system; he had amassed an enormous quantity of knowledge and experience, and his expertise was, quite simply, irreplaceable.[30] Moreover, the reshuffle meant that the other leading international expert, M. D. Perrins, who had shadowed Delevingne's work in Geneva since the early 1920s, would also be transferred away from drugs duties. Perrins' transfer would represent still another loss to the UK's drug control resources.

Anderson's retirement, meanwhile, resulted in the departure of one of only two inspectors working on the domestic aspects, leaving Frank Thornton to monitor the manufacture and wholesale supply of drugs alone. Like the international work, these domestic duties were complex and demanding, necessitating a knowledge of chemical manufacturing processes, the legal framework for control and so forth. All in all, the view at the Home Office was that 'in view of these considerations, we are convinced that there is a risk of serious breakdown' in the drug control functions.[31] These combined developments led to nearly two years of uncertainty and relative chaos for the Home Office staff dealing with drugs. During this period, it was realised that the drugs work was specific and could not be organised along the lines of the regular civil service. Instead, something closer to the previous organisation was required. As Whitelegge reflected: 'Ideally, I suppose, the whole of the drugs work would be operated by a small special Division – along the lines of the "bureaux" in some foreign countries....'[32]

[29] TNA HO 45/24761 'Dangerous Drugs: Organisation of Work', no date.

[30] In fact, an arrangement was made whereby Delevingne stayed on to supervise the international work for a further 18 months. See Ibid.

[31] Ibid.

[32] TNA HO 45/24761, Whitelegge to Harris, 14 July 1933.

By 1933, it had become clear that a more substantial administrative body was required to carry out the range of tasks and meet the UK's international obligations, and the following year, Major William Hewett Coles (who had joined the Home Office in 1924) was appointed to head the new Drugs Branch and Inspectorate.[33] The dispute over staffing arrangements went the way of Delevingne's critics; the Branch's personnel stayed outside the main body of the civil service, did not move across other departments and achieved promotion only within the Drugs Branch. In this way, the necessary expertise was built up over time and remained within the context of the Branch. This remained the case until the 1960s.[34] Delevingne, meanwhile, continued in post at the Drugs Branch for an extra two years, during which he continued to deal with the international dimension of its work, retiring completely from drugs work in 1934.

It was during this period that the newly stabilised Branch began issuing annual reports of its activities. To give a snapshot of its workload, in 1941 the Branch visited approximately 350 licencees (manufactures and wholesalers of drugs) who were inspected annually; the licencees submitted quarterly returns of stocks held and annual reports of their transactions. In addition, the Branch was charged with monitoring 24,000 dentists and 78,000 doctors, chemists and vets authorised under the dangerous drugs regulations, together with some 500 addicts who were investigated and periodically reviewed. It also provided the League of Nations with annual and quarterly reports of UK stocks, manufacture, imports, exports, prosecutions, addiction, raw material requirements and so on.[35]

1933 also saw the formal initiation of the Home Office Addicts Index, which recorded what was supposed to be the UK's total number of addicts, broken down into male and female, therapeutic and nontherapeutic, professional and non-professional. The decision to formalise a central registry from the collection of files that the Drugs Branch had in fact been gathering on addicts since the mid-1920s was prompted by a request from the League of Nations Opium Advisory Committee.[36] However, it must be recalled that the figures were unreliable. This was not least because the

[33] TNA HO 45/24761, HOME OFFICE – STAFF AND OFFICE MATTERS: Pre-war organisation of departmental drugs branch including transfer of obscene publications function (1921–1939).

[34] The staffing arrangements within the interwar Drugs Branch are discussed in: 'Interview 20: Conversation with H.B. Spear' *British Journal of Addiction* 83, (1988), pp. 473–474.

[35] Ibid.

[36] H. B. Spear, *Heroin Addiction, Care and Control* p. 41.

classification as 'therapeutic' or 'nontherapeutic', which appears to be taken as read by many analysts, was highly problematic. Figures such as Brenda Dean Paul and Jean Baird claimed to have become addicted in the course of therapeutic interventions, yet were clearly subcultural addicts—despite their self-representation in the contemporary press. The caveat applies to many of the 1930s and 1940s addicts and renders the early Home Office addiction data at the very least questionable.[37]

The deliberations that took place at the Home Office during the first Brain Committee privately acknowledged this fact. Of the first set of figures that went forward to the League of Nations (which was in 1936), it was observed some 20 years later that 'we do not know ... on what basis the figures ... were compiled'. The author, a Home Office official named Burley, who was advising the secretariat of the first Brain Committee, went on to candidly state that '...much depends on the opinions of the medical advisors and inspectors of the time'.[38] We will have cause to return to this point later in the research, since the Home Office data have been rather too uncritically regarded by researchers; it is sufficient to note here that the statistical information regarding addict numbers compiled by the Home Office and supplied to the League of Nations (and later the United Nations) should be treated as approximate at best. As discussed below, perhaps the most important link in the chain that constructed these data was represented by police inspections of retail pharmacies, and those inspections were of doubtful effectiveness until the early 1960s—particularly in London, which 'cover(ed) about a quarter of the country's population including the majority of the "vicious" addicts'.[39]

Police Inspection of Retail Chemist Shops: A Key Link in the Regulatory Chain

While the Drugs Branch inspectors dealt with licenced organisations that produced and distributed wholesale quantities of dangerous drugs and cases that required 'special inquiry', retail pharmacies were inspected by

[37] The data the Drugs Branch deployed were highly uncertain as a result of the destruction of the Addicts Index in the 1990s, and owing to the fact that it relied upon police inspections of retail pharmacies, which were generally of poor quality, particularly in London where the majority of vicious addicts were located.

[38] TNA HO 391/1, Burley to Goulding, 08.06.1960.

[39] TNA HO 45/ 24,948, Annual Report of Drugs Branch for 1946.

the police. Inspections were carried out twice yearly, usually by detective sergeants. The 1930 Drugs Branch report elaborates on the Branch's functions, and notes that staff should 'regard it as their primary duty to supervise the administration of the Act by the Police'.[40] This supervision would involve systematic visits to forces throughout the country, to ensure that police had adequate staff detailed to dangerous drugs work and that the staff knew what it was doing. Police officers checking pharmacy dangerous drugs records became known as 'Chemist Inspection Officers' (CIOs). 'In view of the impossibility without a large increase in staff of a systematic direct inspection of chemists throughout the country, this is the only practical means of bringing about an effective enforcement of the Act with regard to chemists', wrote the Drugs Branch.[41] The passage states clearly the important role played by police examination of pharmacists' records, and hints at the technical nature of the work and the fact that it would be suitable for the Home Office's own inspectorate were sufficient staff available. Later drug squad officers would remark on the difference between the work carried out by the Home Office, which inspected large companies—who were more likely to observe the regulations—and 'the shabby little chemist in a back street' monitored by police CIOs.[42]

The standard of police retail pharmacy inspection was, however, a continuous source of disquiet at the Drugs Branch and was regarded as generally very weak. The Met's performance, for example, was described by one Drugs Branch inspector as 'poor at the best of times'.[43] There were exceptions to this rule—Glasgow in particular was held up as an 'excellent' example, alongside Manchester and Edinburgh. Why was the general standard of inspection so lacking—particularly given the epistemological and enforcement significance of the task? According to Arthur Kilner, a detective sergeant at Scotland Yard's drug squad writing some decades later, 'between 1921 and about 1962, Police Officers seemed to avoid the task of the inspection of chemist shops, so that if, or when, an inspection was conducted it was done with little knowledge of what was expected of them and frequently with far less enthusiasm'.[44]

[40] TNA HO 45/ 24948, Annual Report of Drugs Branch for 1930.

[41] Ibid.

[42] TNA MEPO 2/10167, Working Party on C.I.D. work in Divisions, Second Interim Report. Dangerous Drugs: Inspection at Chemists' Shops pp. 1–2.

[43] TNA HO45/ 24948, Annual Report of Drugs Branch for 1940.

[44] Shipman Inquiry, 'Guide to Police in Inspection at Chemist Shop' Document GA2600017. No date. http://webarchive.nationalarchives.gov.uk/20090808154959/ http:/www.the-shipman-inquiry.org.uk/reports.asp.

Kilner claims that during this period, little or no training was provided for officers undertaking such inspections and that it was therefore 'a case of "leave well alone"'.[45] This claim is at odds with the surviving annual reports of the Drugs Branch, which, as previously noted, reported making regular visits to police forces to provide appropriate instruction for officers. Either way, it seems certain that there was little taste for the work amongst most officers; it was technical and difficult and involved dealing with middle-class professionals at a time when most police officers were working-class men whose education was often limited to elementary levels. This was despite the fact that police general orders included the reminder that '(s)pecial attention will be paid to the lower-class chemists' shops'.[46] Moreover, chemist shop inspections were not carried out by specialist drugs officers but rather by sergeants who were removed temporarily from their normal case work to undertake the job. There was, consequently, little continuity and scant opportunity to build up the necessary levels of expertise. It was a state of affairs that persisted until the early 1960s, and resulted in cases of opiate prescribing of many years' standing going undetected by the Met's chemist shop inspections, which consequently went unreported to the Home Office until coming to light by chance. It is a matter of speculation as to how many such cases there were before the organisational changes to the policing of drugs took place in 1963.

In fact, the police were most reluctant to take on this work from the beginning. In the context of the Geddes Committee of the early 1920s and the subsequent reductions in public spending, Metropolitan Police Commissioner Horwood wrote to Delevingne as follows: 'The periodic inspection of such (chemists') records in the Metropolis represents the expenditure of a very considerable amount of Police time, and such enquiry as I have made leads me to doubt whether such inspection will be likely to produce any commensurate benefit.'[47] Delevingne, in contrast, argued that police inspections were necessary, and believed that the previous letter indicated that Horwood misunderstood many of the requirements that were to be imposed on the police.[48]

[45] Ibid.

[46] TNA MEPO 2/10167, 'Working Party on CID work in Divisions: Second Interim Report' p. 1.

[47] TNA HO 45/19983, Horwood to Delevingne, 18 July 1922.

[48] TNA HO 45/19983, Delevingne to Horwood, 3 November 1922.

Horwood became still more explicit in his criticism of the proposal: because they lacked the specialised technical training, which was possessed only by chemists, police inspection of pharmacy records 'could only be of a cursory character', and consequently he was 'not satisfied that it would in practice do anything effective towards the prevention of the illegal traffic in drugs'.[49]

Pharmacies were sometimes prosecuted for technical failure to complete records of drugs purchases or prescriptions, and there were occasional cases of deliberate evasion of the regulations and illicit supplies of drugs to addicts. From 1933, retail chemist shops faced additional inspections under the Pharmacy and Poisons Act, carried out by the Pharmaceutical Society of Great Britain (PSGB), their professional regulator. In practice, there was little overlap between the two sets of inspections, except perhaps on an informal basis, as the PSGB had no authority over dangerous drugs.[50] However, Delevingne believed that the letter indicated that Horwood misunderstood many of the requirements that were to be imposed on the police. As usual in these instances of interagency wrangling, Delevingne came out on top, and the regulatory changes duly conferred the Chemist Inspection responsibilities on the police.

Like doctors, pharmacists could have their authority to dispense dangerous drugs withdrawn. According to some, the position was much worse for the pharmacist in this position than for his medical colleague. As one pharmacist wrote in the *Chemist and Druggist* in 1935:

> In the case of the chemist from whom the authorisation to possess or supply has been withdrawn the position under the (National Health Insurance) contract is much more serious. A chemist must dispense the prescriptions brought to him. He has no choice as to the drugs he will supply. He is, therefore, unable to avoid the "dangerous" drugs, and so cannot properly fulfil to dispense insurance prescriptions.

He is also disadvantaged relative to the doctor insofar as 'he cannot engage a deputy to dispense the prescriptions that come under the Dangerous Drugs Acts'.[51]

Doctors whose authority was withdrawn under the Acts were not removed from the National Health Insurance contract, the Ministry of

[49] TNA HO 45/19983, Horwood to Delevingne, 18 July 1922.

[50] H. N. Linstead, *Poisons Law* (London: Pharmaceutical Press, 1936) pp. 204–211.

[51] 'Viator', 'When the D. D. A. Licence is Withdrawn' Chemist *and Druggist* 122, 2883 (1935) p. 572.

Health believing that they could still fulfil their contract, even if it was more difficult to do so. They found ways around the restrictions, such as by having a partner prescribe for their patients.

In the capital, all-night pharmacies such as Boots, located in the Criterion Building at Piccadilly, and John Bell and Croyden in Wigmore Street in the Harley Street medical district played an important dual role. Having opened in the 1920s and early 1930s, they functioned as informal clubs for London's subcultural addicts, who would meet and wait together while their prescriptions were processed—a practice that became the object of tourist 'sightseeing' in the postwar years. A prescription for the next day could be cashed at midnight, and this was consequently a popular time to attend, with queues often forming outside. Simultaneously, these two pharmacies were key sources of data for the Drugs Branch, whose members would often visit, and for the Met, whose Chemist Inspection Officers and specialist drugs investigators were able to extract, both from the pharmacy staff and their records, detailed information about London's addicts.

The Specialist Drugs Work of the Metropolitan Police

Histories of the English police make little or no reference to the use or supply of drugs prior to the Second World War.[52] However, individual drugs officers and small drugs units first arose in the great metropolitan centres, especially London, but also Glasgow, Liverpool, Manchester, Cardiff and others, in response to the sudden growth in newly illicit drug use during and after the First World War. At the passing of the first dangerous drugs legislation, there had been an almost total lack of knowledge amongst the British police concerning the nonmedical use of drugs. The only exception was in respect of opium, which had long been embedded in popular culture and which continued to be smoked in the Chinese communities of Britain's port cities.[53,54] These communities were affected

[52] For example, D. Ascoli, *The Queen's Peace: The Origins and Development of the Metropolitan Police 1829–1979* (London: Hamish Hamilton, 1979).

[53] V. Berridge, (1999) *Opium and the People: Opiate Use and Drug Control Policy in Nineteenth and Early Twentieth Century England* (London: Free Association Books, 1999); T. M. Parssinen, Secret *Passions, Secret Remedies: Narcotic drugs in British Society 1820–1930.* (Philadelphia: Institute for the Study of Human Issues, 1983).

[54] A. Lai; Little, R. & P. Little, 'Chinatown Annie: The East End Opium Trade 1920–35: The Story of a Woman Opium Dealer' *Oral History* 14, 1 (1986) pp. 18–30.

when the 1909 London County Council bye-laws were amended in an attempt to ban opium smoking in Chinese seamen's rooming houses.[55]

The passage of DORA 40B and the 1920 Dangerous Drugs Act was intended to suppress the growth in drug use, and they required enforcing; it was in the course of their enforcement duties that police officers acquired expertise and practical know-how regarding dangerous drugs and those who consumed them. In addition to acquainting themselves with the new legislation, they learned (to a degree that varied greatly) to recognise substances, states of intoxication, codes and signs used by formative drug subcultures, the characteristic spaces frequented by these groups and so on. While the officers were not formally designated as drug specialists in the public statements of the police, in practice some of them became such; others were given specialist roles on a more or less ad hoc basis. Perhaps the first of the specialist officers was Walter Burmby, born in London in 1879, who became a detective sergeant and then an inspector based in the Scotland Yard headquarters of the Met. Burmby was the leading investigator and arresting officer in numerous well-known drug cases such as that of Edgar Manning, the actress Cissie Loftus, the opium traffickers Albert Ellis and May Roberts, the prescription frauds of morphine addicts Patrick and Winifred McKay as well as those of several doctors.[56,57,58,59] Often assisted by Constable Charles Owen, Burmby worked on drug cases throughout the 1920s, and his promotion to divisional inspector in 1929 prompted comment by *The Times*, which reported that he had 'been for years the special officer in charge of investigations in connection with the drug traffic'.[60]

In the early 1930s, Edward Griffey took on this role, having worked as a constable in the early 1920s with Sergeant Goddard at the Vine Street Clubs Office, the same George Goddard who would later face corruption charges and made a handsome living from the payments he received from nightclub proprietors such as the celebrated Irene Meyrick.[61] By the early

[55] V. Berridge, 'East End Opium Dens and Narcotic Use in Britain' *The London Journal*, 4, 1 (1978) pp. 3–20.

[56] M. Kohn, *Dope Girls*, pp. 154–158.

[57] *Times* 11 November 1922, p. 7.

[58] *Times* 8 January 1923, p. 7.

[59] *Times* 27 August 1924, p. 7.

[60] *Times* 2 August 1929, p. 14.

[61] J. Walkowitz (2012) *Nights Out: Life in Cosmopolitan London* Yale University Press (Chap. 7).

1930s, Griffey was doing regular work on drug cases and played a prominent part in the investigation and arrests of Brenda Dean Paul and Anthea Carew. He was also involved in large-scale trafficking cases such as that of Deeble, Cole and McCain, moving opium and cocaine between Montreal, Antwerp and London; the heroin addict and suicide Barbara Gamble; and the later, abortionist phase of the career of Dr Connor.[62,63] During the 1939–45 war, Sergeant (later Inspector) Garrod of New Scotland Yard CID handled many of the force's drug cases.[64] He would later lecture on dangerous drugs at the Met's training college at Hendon.[65]

The Metropolitan Police drug squad was established as a formally designated entity in 1954.[66] However, prior to this, there was a drugs office at New Scotland Yard, formed shortly after the end of the Second World War, with a reshuffle of resources resulting in the 'practical creation of a small "Drug Squad"'.[67] One detective sergeant was principally occupied with drugs work, and two more were made available to assist as required. The key officer was George Lyle, who worked in close contact with the Drugs Branch; Harry 'Chips' Carpenter was his usual assistant. Having moved from his native Scotland to the capital to join the Met in 1936, Lyle fought in the RAF during the Second World War, returning to his police duties following the end of hostilities. Lyle was involved with drugs work for most of the remainder of his career; according to his daughter, he would commute from their home in Surbiton each day equipped with bowler hat and umbrella.[68] She also tells how he was approached by Maureen Guinness (of the brewing family) with regard to her daughter Caroline, who married and later divorced the painter Lucian Freud and was a regular at the Gargoyle Club, run by David Tennant.[69] In later years

[62] TNA HO 144/22433 DANGEROUS DRUGS AND POISONS: Trafficking: first case of joint police action with other countries effecting simultaneous arrests in London, Montreal and Antwerp, 1932–1943.

[63] *Daily Mail* 31 August 1932, p. 5; *Times* 31 August 1932, p. 7.

[64] See TNA MEPO 3/2579.

[65] See TNA MEPO 2/9631 Dangerous Drugs: Trafficking, Prosecution, Inspection, Lectures, 1954–1955.

[66] J. H. Mills, Cannabis *Nation* p. 129. See also TNA MEPO 2/10167 CID to Home Office 11 February 1972. The file makes clear that 1954 was the point at which two or more police officers were first assigned to full-time drugs work.

[67] TNA HO 45/24948, Annual Report of the Home Office Drugs Branch for 1947.

[68] *Daily Record* 31 July 2012, http://www.dailyrecord.co.uk/news/real-life/special-drugs-unit-became-standard-1196680. Accessed 60.09.2012.

[69] See Chap. 3 of this book.

she was better known as the writer Caroline Blackwood.[70] Guinness explained that she was anxious about her daughter's drug use—though in due course Caroline would settle on alcohol as her drug of choice—and asked Lyle to help; he advised her, however, that in his view a 'talking-to' from a policeman was unlikely to make much difference.[71] What remained as a historical continuity here was the reticence of London's police to interfere with the illicit pleasures of the upper classes unless and until they openly flouted the law, as in the case of Brenda Dean Paul, Anthea Carew and their set.

It is significant that Detective Sergeant Arthur Leonard Dyke, known as 'Len' Dyke, who was Lyle's immediate predecessor as the Met's expert drugs officer, had moved across to join the Drugs Branch during 1941 when the demands of war had drastically reduced staff numbers, so that at one point the Branch consisted solely of Frank Thornton, its chief inspector. Dyke was intimately acquainted with the West End and was at the forefront in the arrest of both Bella Gold and Freda Roberts, associates of Gerry O'Brien, the heroin user and supplier and a well-known figure in the West End life.[72] Dyke had also been a Chemist Inspection Officer for the Met, developing a range and degree of expertise that made his transfer to the Drugs Branch imperative for the Branch at a time when it was denuded of most of its resources. His transfer brought still closer the links between the Branch and the Met's drugs officers. Something of a moral crusader against the growing drug subculture, Dyke 'took every new addict as a personal defeat' and went on to become the Drugs Branch chief inspector between 1956 and 1964.[73] He was to be a key figure during the last decade of the classic British System; his police background and strong moral perspective regarding drugs seems to have ushered in a more punitive focus at the Branch, against a background of rising drug consumption, youth culture and scepticism toward authority figures of all kinds.

[70] N. Schoenberger *Dangerous Muse: The Life of Lady Caroline Blackwood* (New York: Da Capo Press, 2001).

[71] *Daily Record* 31 July 2012.

[72] This group is discussed in detail in Chap. 5.

[73] 'Conversation with Bing Spear: Journal Interview 20', *British Journal of Addiction* 83 (1988) p. 475.

Drugs, Clubs and Corruption in the Metropolitan Police 'C' Division

Many of the capital's drug cases in the interwar years were dealt with by the central London divisions, especially 'C' Division, which mapped onto the administrative area of St James, and included both Soho and Mayfair.[74] During the 1930s, 'C' Division was served by two stations, Vine Street and Great Marlborough Street, each of which was attached to a police court, known today as magistrates' courts.[75] An early Met unit whose work included a familiarity with the drug scene was the Clubs Office, a specialist department based at Vine Street station that was popularly named the 'vice squad' after its American counterparts. Established in 1932, the Clubs Office dealt with 'vice' in the West End, London's pleasure district, focusing on commercial sex transactions, nightclubs, bottle parties and licencing infringements; the milieu in which the unit operated also brought it into close proximity with the users and suppliers of drugs. As noted above, it was at Vine Street that Sergeant George Goddard was stationed, and where clubs-related duties involved officers in close relationships with criminal networks, allowing them direct and continuous exposure to the potential for bribery and corruption.

In Goddard's instance, it was a potential that was realised on a fairly grand scale. The authorities had long denied any suggestion of corruption amongst police officers, the Marlborough Street magistrate Frederick Mead, for example, telling the parliamentary Street Offences Committee in 1927 that popular belief in the bribery of police for money or sex from prostitutes arose due to men—members of the public—impersonating officers and promising not to arrest them if they provided payment in money or sex.[76] However, the exposure of Goddard's activities threatened to shatter the myth of the incorruptible English constable.

George Goddard was a former bricklayer and had joined the police in 1900. He was exonerated on charges of corruption by a 1922 inquiry but in 1928 was finally dismissed from the police for accepting bribes and

[74] The others were 'A' Division, which included Westminster and Whitehall and in which the original Met headquarters at Scotland Yard was located; 'B' Division, Chelsea; 'D' Division, Marylebone; 'E' Division, Holborn; and 'F' division, Paddington.

[75] West End Central Station in Savile Row was opened in 1940 to replace these two stations. See M. Fido and K. Skinner, *The Official Encyclopaedia of Scotland Yard* (London: Virgin Books, 1999) p. 283.

[76] *Times* 3 December 1927, p. 4.

consorting with nightclub owners, including Kate Meyrick, and operators of brothels.[77] In receipt of some £6.15 per week wages, the sergeant had accumulated assets worth £18,000. The case was, as Emsley notes, represented as exceptional, a 'bad apple'. However, the commissioner's report for 1931 referred to the 'highly unsatisfactory state of affairs on the Great Marlborough Street section of "C" Division', as a result of which disciplinary action was taken against an inspector, 2 section sergeants and 40 constables. Twenty-seven of the men were dismissed, including the inspector.[78] Emsley adds that a further 24 men, including at least 1 inspector, were transferred to other divisions in the aftermath of the affair.[79] This was a major shake-up by any standards and demonstrated the corruption that was rife in 'C' Division at the time of the Goddard affair.

The frequenting of known criminal haunts was accepted as a part of the working method of detectives. According to historian Stefan Petrow, the use of paid informants became widespread in the 1870s, and at the end of the nineteenth century, informants had become 'the base of detective duty'.[80] This was particularly true for specialist units like the Clubs Office. It emerged during the trial of Kate Meyrick and restaurateur Luigi Ribuffi for bribing Goddard that amongst those from whom the sergeant had been receiving payments was Jack May, proprietor of Murray's Club in Beak Street. May was one of the figures embroiled in the Billie Carleton affair after the actress died of a supposed cocaine overdose in 1918.[81] He was alleged to have introduced young women including Carleton to cocaine and to the practice of opium smoking and to have supplied cocaine from his clubs in London and Maidenhead.[82] While the trial concentrated on payments Goddard was able to extract to ensure that the Met would not interfere with the smooth running of the nightclubs and brothels of Soho, the inclusion of no less a figure than Jack May raises the distinct

[77] C. Emsley, 'Sergeant Goddard: the story of a rotten apple or a diseased orchard?' in A. G. Srebnik & R. Levy, (eds) *Crime and culture: an historical perspective* (Advances in Criminology. Aldershot: Ashgate, 2005) pp. 85–104.

[78] *Report of the Commissioner of the Metropolitan Police for the Year 1931* London: HMSO p. 7.

[79] C. Emsley, *The Great British Bobby: A History of British Policing from the 18th Century to the Present* (London: Quercus, 2009) p. 206.

[80] S. Petrow, *Policing Morals: The Metropolitan Police and the Home Office, 1870–1914* (Oxford: Clarendon Press, 1994) p. 57.

[81] M. Kohn, *Dope Girls*, p. 32, *passim*.

[82] M. Sweet, *Shepperton Babylon: The Lost Worlds of British Cinema* (London: Faber and Faber, 2006) pp. 47–50.

possibility that drug suppliers too participated in 'C' Division's system of kickbacks.

The close involvement of police officers with the milieu in which drugs moved in the West End, especially where criminal subcultures overlapped with the night-time economy and its pleasures, probably meant some degree of corruption was inevitable; we should not be surprised. It is interesting, though, to observe the involvement of the drug trade with the paying off of law enforcement agents at this early point in the history of London's illicit market. It was not only the police who were exposed to such risks; while there is no evidence of corruption, the Drugs Branch inspectors too engaged in a peripatetic style of knowledge-building that saw them visiting clubs and parties on the West End scene, crossing cultural boundaries in order to gather drugs intelligence at first hand. Spear reported in an interview in the 1980s that Frank Thornton and Len Dyke, who was in the 1930s still a policeman, conducted these types of forays into the West End. Such practices were already underway during 'that period just before the war when there was a little upper-crust heroin circle which he (Dyke) and Thornton knew quite well'.[83] Spear also wrote of Dyke's and Thornton's information gathering trips in the West End and that Thornton 'was a member of some of the well-known clubs, though not everyone was convinced he had joined them, as he always claimed, to gather intelligence'.[84] Spear himself was later widely known for his friendly relations with West End addicts, recalling that: 'If things were slow in the office, I'd say, "I'll put my coat on and go to Boots and John Bell and Croyden (the chemists) for the afternoon".'[85] There he would examine the dangerous drugs registers, as well as meeting addicts who called in to cash their prescriptions. Sarah Mars, meanwhile, tells us that in the early 1960s when Charles Jeffery was chief inspector at the Branch, 'drug users often invited themselves for tea' at the Home Office.[86]

As observed by Emsley, the experiential knowledge of the criminal and his haunts is a standard trope of the police memoir; nonetheless, it was a vital element in the dance of addicts and regulators in days of the classic

[83] 'Conversation with Bing Spear: Journal Interview 20', *British Journal of Addiction* 83, (1988) p. 473.

[84] H. B. Spear, *Heroin Addiction, Care and Control* p. 59.

[85] 'Conversation with Bing Spear: Journal Interview 20', *British Journal of Addiction* (1988) 83, p. 474.

[86] S. Mars, *Politics of Addiction*, p. 92.

British System.[87] Many of London's drug users and police officers knew each other by sight and often by name in this tight, localised scene.[88] Beyond this, if unknown to one another, they learned to recognise clues of dress, posture, haircut and speech patterns: each side knew this and adapted their clothing and deportment in an attempt to evade the gaze of the other. The commercial sex scene, which was interlinked closely with that of drugs, also provided a key source of intelligence for the police.[89]

Medical Regulation of Addiction

The investigation of doctors was shared between the Drugs Branch and the Ministry of Health, whose RMOs played a role in dealing with practitioners whose prescribing or purchases of drugs drew regulatory attention.[90] Mars' statement that '(by) the 1920s it was not the Home Office Inspectors or the police who inspected the supply of dangerous drugs but medical officials' appears to rest on a misunderstanding.[91] RMOs would undertake a limited amount of routine inspections of doctors' records, but the dangerous drugs records at retail pharmacies were inspected by the police, and any discrepancies observed in doctors' prescriptions (long-term or high-dose prescribing, cases of dual supply, etc.) were passed on to the Drugs Branch. If the Branch judged that the prescribing doctor was likely to be supplying an addict, or was himself an addict, the arrangement with the RMO service would then kick in, and the doctor in question would be visited.

The Regional Medical Service was assigned this authority under the dangerous drugs regulations in 1922; at the same time, it was agreed by the Ministry that RMOs would carry out routine inspections of doctors' records on a periodic basis.[92] RMOs did not possess the authority to force doctors to change their methods of treating addiction—these remained within the sovereign professional domain of the practitioner, which, despite the encroachments of the state around the dangerous drugs issue,

[87] C. Emsley, *Crime and Society* pp. 131–136.

[88] M. Kohn, 'Life and Times: Grains of Truth' *The Guardian*, September 1st 1990.

[89] J. Laite, *Common Prostitutes and Ordinary Citizens: Commercial Sex in London, 1885–1960* (Basingstoke: Palgrave Macmillan, 2011) p. 141; see also H. Daley, (1986) *This Small Cloud: A Personal Memoir* (London: Weidenfeld & Nicholson, 1986) pp. 148,159,164.

[90] TNA HO45/ 24948, Annual Report of Drugs Branch for 1930; Memo of 28.03.1930.

[91] S. Mars, *The Politics of Addiction* p. 91.

[92] TNA HO 45/19983, Ministry of Health to Home Office 10 November 1922.

continued to be effectively defended by the profession and its allies. Nonetheless, it seems clear that informal pressures were at times exerted on prescribing practitioners by both RMOs and Drugs Branch inspectors.

Historically, the suggestion to use RMOs in this capacity came first from the Ministry. The Home Office had observed that the use of police officers to inspect the records of doctors would not be desirable, and its reservations were made known to the Ministry, which agreed. It suggested that, as the national insurance records of practitioners were already being inspected by RMOs, it would be simple and advantageous to extend their duties to include the inspection of dangerous drugs records.[93]

The precise arrangements were negotiated between the two government departments. The Home Office wondered, 'Could your inspectors in the course of their inspections say whether doctors are prescribing or dispensing the drugs excessively?'[94] The Ministry of Health, meanwhile, was keen to downplay such expectations. It pointed out that RMOs were not authorised under the Acts to carry out inspections of prescriptions, of which only dispensing doctors kept copies anyway. These were the responsibility of the police. With regard to the monitoring of excess by prescribing physicians, it argued that 'in most cases ... this would be very difficult since there are wide variations in the quantities of these drugs which different doctors would quite legitimately order for their patients. Some doctors for instance order far more opium than others'.[95]

There was a considerable groundswell of opinion against the allocation of these duties to RMOs. Alfred Cox and the British Medical Association were against it from the beginning. 'I suppose it was inevitable in the present stage of the cultivation of the economy hobby', he wrote, 'but to my mind it is a bad business.' Cox argued that RMOs were already overworked and that the new dangerous drugs duties would 'be the last straw for some of them'. More importantly, though, was that it 'emphasised the official and, if I may call it so, the detective side of their duties to the grave disadvantage of the far more important advisory side'. These officers performed regular checks on the national insurance work of doctors and were already viewed by some with suspicion. But their appearance in the role of

[93] TNA HO 45/19983, Ministry of Health to Home Office 18 October 1921.
[94] TNA HO 45/19983, Kirwan to McCleary, 7 September 1922.
[95] TNA HO 45/19983, McCleary to Kirwan, 23 September 1922.

Home Office inspectors would, said Cox, 'damn them effectively in the eyes of a considerable section of the profession'.[96]

It is, however, difficult to estimate how prevalent Cox's views were. Delevingne sent Cox's letter to McCleary at the Ministry, who did 'not share the pessimistic forebodings' expressed. McCleary further believed that 'working on the lines we have mutually agreed the inspections should enhance rather than impair the position of the Regional staff in relation to the Medical profession generally'.[97] If there was unease amongst the Regional Medical Service at its dangerous drugs tasks, the Drugs Branch at times expressed less than flattering opinions of RMOs. As 'Len' Dyke commented on the role of RMOs and their relations with Home Office inspectors:

> Successful interrogation of any doctor suspected of addiction, offences, etc., is acquired only by practice and initiative, a "curious" turn of mind, the tendency not to always accept *no* for an answer and so on; to this one must add a thorough knowledge of Dangerous Drugs laws. I fear these points and other relevant aspects are normally beyond the average RMO.

The degree to which these opinions were shared is, once again, difficult to gauge.

In addition to providing them with a letter to act as warrant of their authority to carry out these inspections, the Ministry of Health produced detailed instructions for its RMOs when their new inspection duties commenced in 1923. These were organised under two headings, 'routine' and 'special' inspections. The former referred only to doctors who dispensed their own medicines, as those who did not were at this stage not obliged by the legislation to keep records. This meant that most doctors were not subject to routine visits by RMOs. Any suspicions were not acted upon by the RMO but reported to the Home Office which took the decision as to what, if any, action should be taken. Routine inspections were, moreover, carried out only in England and Wales; the Scottish Board of Health restricted RMOs to visits in exceptional circumstances. Special inspections took place when the Home Office requested the RMO to visit a practitioner, with instructions issued to the officer on a case-by-case basis. These were usually examples in which the Home Office suspected the possibility of addiction, either of the practitioner or a patient, which was being supplied with drugs in contravention to the law.

[96] TNA HO 45/19983, Cox to Delevingne, 1 February 1923.
[97] TNA HO 45/19983, McCleary to Delevingne, 4 February 1923.

It is important to recognise that in this context much of the regulatory pressure was exerted by one part of the regulatory system on another. As we have seen, doctors were permitted to provide supplies of drugs for addicts in certain cases; this was itself a regulatory measure, securing the addict within a medical system of observation and record-keeping and theoretically maintaining doses at low levels. RMOs were called in by the Home Office to investigate in those circumstances where it appeared that doctors were not following the regulations governing such supplies. It was felt that 'medical men' were more suited to discussion of the complexities arising from cases of treatment than the Drugs Branch's inspectors, and the Ministry of Health was assured that no medical professional would be placed in the invidious position of having to give evidence against a colleague in a court of law.[98] Nevertheless, within a few years of the establishment of this arrangement, Dr Dill Russell, an RMO who regularly worked in cases of transgressive prescribing, was called as a witness for the prosecution in the case against Dr George Kingsbury, who had refused to supply the Home Office with the name of an addict patient. Dr Kingsbury was motivated, he protested, by a concern for his patient's confidentiality and was fined.[99]

The main object of Drugs Branch attentions was the script doctor, who was viewed as the primary source of addiction when his prescribing or administration of dangerous drugs went beyond the informal limits that were supposed to be guaranteed by the system. Where it felt it necessary, the Home Office made use of the testimony of RMOs to obtain legal or professional restrictions on the prescribing of the transgressive practitioner.

The Regional Medical Service was suspended during the Second World War, and the impact upon the work of the Drugs Branch was considerable.[100] The Branch was operating on very short staff during wartime, and its inspectors were now required to undertake the visits to doctors previously carried out by the RMOs. S. J. Sloane, the inspector who drafted the

[98] See TNA HO 144/11969 Dangerous Drugs and Poisons: Interpretation of Regulation 4 of Dangerous Drugs Regulations, 1921: the case stated against Dr George Chadwick Kingsbury.

[99] *Times* 2 March 1926, p. 6; *Times* 11 November 1926, p. 5.

[100] In the months preceding the war while the Emergency Medical Service was being established, the Home Office reported that 'the Ministry of Health have completely dropped their routines visits of inspection, and even special visits of inspection at our request'. TNA HO 45/24948, Annual Report of the Drugs Branch for 1939.

Branch's Annual Report for 1940, complained that his visits to doctors had increased from 38 in 1939 to 114 in 1940, an increase of around 300 per cent.[101] Sloane stated moreover that 'these visits are highly wasteful of inspection time owing to the difficulty of seeing doctors and involve, in some cases, two visits before they can be seen'.[102] This was due to the doctors' appointment schedules, home visits and so forth—they were hard to pin down, even in circumstances where nothing illicit was involved, and more so when it was. In addition, the text notes that script doctors 'produce far more difficulties than in dealing with the out-and-out addict doctor, or one who is suspected of addiction'.[103] This was, presumably, due to the problems of obtaining proof thrown up by such cases.

Aside from RMOs, there were two other main medical structures involved in the regulatory endeavour. First was the General Medical Council ('GMC' or 'Council'), to which Dr Reginald Nitch Smith had been referred by the husband of his patient Deborah Platt, following on from the highly critical remarks by the Old Bailey judge who heard her case and who recommended that the doctor should be professionally disciplined.[104] Nitch Smith was subsequently found guilty of infamous conduct in a professional respect and struck off the register by the Council.[105] However, after this episode the GMC was generally reluctant to hear such cases except when the practitioner had already been found guilty of an offence under the law.[106] The Home Office was, in its turn, unwilling to make use of the tribunal system that the Rolleston Committee had provided as an essential part of the control machinery for handling script doctors. The tribunal, composed of medical personnel supported by a legal advisor, was designed to enable 'overprescribing' physicians to be prevented from supplying dangerous drugs without the necessity of a criminal case.[107] Home Office reluctance to make use of the mechanism led to continuing problems in the regulation of prescribing doctors. The preferred method continued to be that of securing a conviction under the

[101] TNA HO 45/24948, Annual Report of the Drugs Branch for 1940.

[102] Ibid.

[103] Ibid.

[104] *British Medical Journal* 2, 2971, (1917) pp. 113–115.

[105] Ibid.

[106] S. Mars, *The Politics of Addiction* p. 67.

[107] P. Bean, 'Policing the Medical Profession: The Use of Tribunals' in D. K. Whynes & P. Bean (eds) *Policing and Prescribing: The British System of Drug Control* (Basingstoke, Hampshire: Macmillan, 1991) pp. 60–70.

Dangerous Drugs Acts, and the subsequent removal by the secretary of state of the doctor's authority to prescribe and dispense drugs.[108] As has already been demonstrated, such tactics were by no means universally effective. Those practitioners who managed to avoid prosecution could not have their authority withdrawn in this way and were consequently able to continue their practices with relative impunity.

This chapter has illustrated the development of the early, ad hoc drug control architecture into formal mechanisms. It is notable that the retirement of a single individual, Sir Malcolm Delevingne, played a central role in both the near collapse of the Home Office structures and their subsequent rebuilding through necessity. Generally, however, the boundaries between the various components of the regime—international and domestic, police and medical—showed a strong tendency to blur the lines of demarcation that were supposed to divide them. Indeed, much of the regime's regulatory energy went toward policing itself.

[108] H. B. Spear, *Heroin Addiction, Care and Control* pp. 45–48.

CHAPTER 6

The Royal College of Physicians Committee on Drug Addiction, c.1938–c.1947

Introduction

The preceding chapters have demonstrated the ways in which the vicious addicts of the 1930s adapted to the regulatory framework that sought to govern and restrict their use of morphine, heroin and cocaine. The West End network moved around the restrictions, sourcing illicit drugs directly from suppliers in Paris. The Chelsea network, meanwhile, made use of the restrictive system, obtaining their supplies from doctors who were themselves often viewed as transgressors and yet were an essential part of the regulatory apparatus. Thus, despite the legislative and regulatory architecture surrounding it, the nonmedical use of what were supposed to be controlled drugs continued. This chapter explores the discontent provoked by this state of affairs at the time amongst pockets of the medical profession—particularly specialists in addiction. The specific focus is on the 1938 Royal College of Physicians Committee on Drug Addiction, established to examine the problem of addiction, its treatment and the control machinery that surrounded it. The Committee formed the centre of the profession's pervasive unease at the way in which the Rolleston regulations had been applied in practice. There was a powerful eugenic strand in the Committee's makeup, an element that had long been associated with a trend toward the incarceration of addicts and which peaked in the interwar period. Eugenics was tightly associated with the concept of inebriety and with the legislation devised to confine inebriates in hybrid

C. Hallam, *White Drug Cultures and Regulation in London, 1916–1960*, https://doi.org/10.1007/978-3-319-94770-9_6

carceral spaces under the aegis of medicine.[1] It was the eugenics movement that provided the initial impetus for the RCP to conduct its review.

There was tactical spilt between two factions on the Committee that revolved around the question of whether compulsory detention should be applied to addicts alone or to the deviant population more broadly. The more ambitious eugenicist strand was grouped around the king's physician, Lord Dawson of Penn, and sought to expand the Committee's terms of reference to allow for the broader objective. Meanwhile the other major faction, with Dr Russell Brain at its centre, was anxious that such a policy could alienate the government and the legal profession, thereby preventing the attainment of both the wider eugenic objective and the more limited goal of confining those addicted to dangerous drugs. In the event, the dissent on the Committee prevented it from exerting any decisive influence on policy-makers, though the objective of placing addicts in preventive detention in state-funded homes was briefly revived by the Home Office in the immediate postwar period, for reasons that will be made clear below. Less ambitious forms of compulsion would also reappear in the second report of the Brain Committee, published in 1965, of which Russell Brain was the chair and which recommended that its proposed treatment centres be permitted to compulsorily detain addicts during periods of crisis associated with opiate withdrawal. The recommendation, which the Committee acknowledged would require new legislation, was not acted upon. Nonetheless, the principle of compulsion has in various forms retained its place in the discussion of addiction policies, and continues to be invoked periodically into the present day.

The documentation produced by the RCP Committee provides a revealing insight into the views of some of the most influential figures amongst the elite of the interwar medical profession regarding addiction medicine in general and the performance of the British System in particular. There has been surprisingly little academic research on the RCP Committee and its work, with only sociologist Carol Smart offering a sustained analysis. Her argument touches on the concepts of eugenics, but its central objective is to explore the principle of medicalisation; essentially, it uses the ideas of Michel Foucault to trace the problematic figure of the addict in the context of the disciplinary society, and the obligation to

[1] H. Padwa, *Social Poison: The Culture and Politics of Opiate Control in Britain and France, 1891–1926*. (Baltimore: Johns Hopkins University Press, 2012) pp. 34, 35, 149.

health and rationality it imposes.[2] A few other researchers, such as Virginia Berridge, mention the RCP Committee briefly; importantly, Berridge notes the link it provides with both the inebriates legislation of the late Victorian and Edwardian era and the recommendations of the postwar Brain Committees.[3]

Background

The will to sequester and confine drug addicts was not a new one and was intimately bound up with the eugenicist project of racial improvement. As Berridge notes of late nineteenth-century Britain: 'The eugenic influence in general scientific thinking and in the disease theory (of addiction) in particular, brought with it a trend toward compulsory segregation, also manifested in the continuing contemporary discussion of the forcible segregation in labour colonies of the unemployed and the "undeserving poor".'[4] Since the emergence of the discourse of inebriety toward the end of the Victorian age, there had been tensions regarding the use of compulsion and confinement amongst those seeking to establish a medical vocabulary and procedures in relation to addiction.

Carceral responses were advocated particularly when the inebriate came from the lower strata of society. Under the inebriates legislation of 1898, habitual drunkards could be subjected to confinement in state-funded institutions, but this was conditional upon convictions for drunkenness. The Inebriates Acts extended beyond alcohol to the use of other types of intoxicants, but only if the latter were imbibed: the smoking or injecting of a substance was excluded from their application, and in practice, these laws were rarely applied in cases of drug addiction.[5] From the 1880s, many doctors advocated compulsory commitment under the Inebriates Acts. In cooperation with the Society for the Study of Inebriety, the British Medical Association set up an Inebriates Legislation Committee to lobby for such changes; Norman Kerr, the leading British exponent of a disease model of addiction, provided the key link between these networks, being a leading light in both. However, their activism was unsuccessful; the legislation

[2] C. Smart, 'Social Policy and Drug Addiction: A Critical Study of Policy Development' *British Journal of Addiction* 79, (1984) pp. 31–39.

[3] Berridge, *Opium and the People*, p. 181.

[4] Berridge, *Opium and the People*, p. 165.

[5] V. Berridge, 'Punishment or Treatment? Inebriety, Drink, and Drugs 1860–2004', *The Lancet* Special Issue: Medicine, Crime and Punishment. Volume 364, (2004).

they sought was not enacted, and relatively few addicts were confined in prison or lunatic asylums. In the early twentieth century, the Acts fell steadily into disuse, but the question of confinement remained alive in debates around the handling of drug addicts and re-emerged as a central theme in the context of the RCP Committee.

The antipathy toward maintenance and long-term prescribing attached itself to this discourse. As pointed out by Alex Mold, there were many doctors on the Rolleston Committee and in the British medical profession generally who were opposed—some strongly—to the provision of maintenance doses.[6] After Rolleston's recommendations were incorporated into state drug policy, these physicians remained dissatisfied with contemporary therapeutic practice toward addicts, and continued to advocate rapid withdrawal, compulsion and institutional confinement.

The debate over addiction treatment was also kept alive in the courts when widely reported cases of addiction came before them. The Brenda Dean Paul and Anthea Carew cases led the Home Office to speculate that:

> What is wanted is a power to commit to an approved institution where the addict will receive proper treatment (and proper treatment includes not only the elimination of the craving but also the after-care for building up the patient physically and morally) and which the addict will not be allowed to leave except under licence. I believe magistrates would welcome a provision of this kind, which would greatly simplify their task.[7]

Such observations were, in addition, regularly made by magistrates themselves and were debated in the expert medical press.[8,9]

The Eugenics Movement and the Initiative for the RCP Committee

Eugenics was essentially a project of racial management—a biological politics—and its objective was to improve the quality of the race. The eugenics programme set out to increase the numbers of well-born, superior racial

[6] Mold, (2008) *Heroin*, pp. 18–20.

[7] TNA MH 135/157, 'Dangerous Drugs- Withdrawal of authority to prescribe'. Notes on the control and cure of drug addicts. n.d.

[8] *Daily Express* 13 March 1931, p. 7.

[9] 'Medicine and the Law: Prison or Hospital for Drug Addict?' *Lancet* 232, 5999 (1938), pp. 454–455. The discussion was prompted by the Patricia Mallory court case; see Chap. 5.

stock and to apply birth control to the lower orders, large numbers of whom were viewed as a 'standing army of biological misfits'.[10] The 'population panic' of the 1930s centred on the perceived degrading of Britain's racial heritage, and it was feared that the lower orders of the population were reproducing in vast numbers, while the superior elements failed to keep procreative pace; the use of contraception and the selfishness of the middle-class woman, who was felt to be obsessed with pleasure and consumption, were often blamed for this state of affairs.[11] The eugenic concern in the RCP Committee lay with the entire biopolitical class of the social problem group or the 'unfit', in which addicts were included. Control over addicts, it was felt, offered a way into to the larger eugenic project of reducing the numbers of the unfit.

Although eugenics is often regarded as reaching its peak in the Edwardian period, according to Richard Overy, 'the high point of the British eugenics movement, and of eugenics internationally, came in the years between the two world wars'.[12] In Britain, the movement was influential in provoking and articulating public anxieties, issuing in government committees of inquiry into population policy, the 'feeble-minded', syphilis, alcoholism, drug addiction and so on (Humphrey Rolleston was himself a member of the Eugenics Society). These investigations took place against the backdrop of an intellectual climate of impending disaster, a sense of what Overy calls 'biological catastrophe' that pervaded the 1930s, and one can clearly see these anxious thematics at work on the RCP Committee.[13]

The National Council for Mental Hygiene (NCMH) was formed in 1922 in a meeting held at the Royal Society of Medicine in Wimpole Street, attended by numerous dignitaries from medicine, science and politics. Its aim was to improve the prevention and treatment of mental disorder.[14] The NCMH was part of a spread of eugenicist organisations and possessed an abiding interest in drug addicts and addiction. Dr R. D.

[10] Eugenics Review, quoted in J. Gardiner, *Wartime: Britain 1939–1945* (London: Headline, 2004) p. 214.

[11] P. Thane, (1995) 'Population Politics in Post-War British Culture' in R. Conekin, F. Mort, Frank & C. Waters, (eds.) *Moments of Modernity: Reconstructing Britain 1945–1964* (London & New York: Rivers Oram Press, 1999) pp. 114–133.

[12] Overy, *The Morbid Age*, p. 105.

[13] Ibid., p. 107.

[14] *Times*, 5 May 1922, p. 18. Among the speakers was Humphrey Rolleston, then president of the RCP, and those present included Sir George Newman, principal medical officer at the

Gillespie, honorary secretary to the NCMH, was quoted in 1933 to the effect that 'the present custom of allowing drug addicts to live in the outside world with a permitted daily allowance of morphia is repugnant to the medical mind'.[15] Gillespie believed that addicts, alcoholics, homosexuals ('perverts') and failed suicides should all be confined. Like his colleague Dr Hugh Crichton-Miller, Gillespie was a member of both the RCP and the NCMH; it was these two men who initiated the process from which the RCP Committee was to emerge.

In 1938, the RCP was approached by Crichton-Miller on behalf of the NCMH, 'asking the College for its cooperation in seeking to secure further legislative powers to secure efficient treatment in drug addicts' (sic). The RCP Comitia—essentially the general assembly of the RCP—approved the proposal.[16] The formal motion was made by Gillespie, who told the College that 'it was well-known that the present method of dealing with drug addicts was a failure and that relapses were extremely common'. He went on to explain that the 'fundamental fallacy' of the voluntary method of addiction treatment was that it assumed possession of will power when the condition in question was marked precisely by a failure of volition. It was time, Gillespie argued, to consider the adoption of 'more definite powers' in dealing with addicts and alcoholics. The motion was seconded, and the president would nominate a suitable committee to consider the issue.[17]

The Composition of the RCP Committee on Drug Addiction

The RCP Committee on Drug Addiction held a series of eight meetings throughout 1938, in addition to various subsidiary sessions. The discussions took place at the RCP's headquarters in Pall Mall East, overlooking Trafalgar Square and close to the government district of Whitehall. Here, the nonmedical uses of drugs were understood purely in terms of pathology and of crime. The Royal College was one of the core institutions on the elite side of the divide running through British medicine, and the

Ministry of Health; C. H. Bond, president of the British Medico-Psychological Association; Lord Dawson of Penn; and several MPs.

[15] *Gloucestershire Echo* 25 November 1933, p. 1.

[16] Archive of the Royal College of Physicians. Official Proceedings of the Royal College of Physicians, 1935–1937; Volume LVI p. 393.

[17] Official Proceedings of the Royal College of Physicians, 1935–1937; Volume LVI p. 503.

Committee on Drug Addiction was composed of ten individuals, nine of whom were men and amongst the most eminent figures in the 1930s medical landscape.[18]

Dr Bernard Hart was the Committee's chairman, one of the early physicians working with the 'shellshock' concept during the Great War and the author of a highly popular contemporary textbook on psychopathology.[19] He was joined by the royal physician Bertrand Dawson (Viscount Dawson of Penn), who had in 1928 achieved national celebrity by saving the life of George V, and had in 1936 hastened the demise of the same monarch through a timely injection of heroin and cocaine into the royal jugular.[20] Penn was president of the RCP from 1931 to 1937; he was joined on the Committee by Sir William Willcox, expert in addiction medicine and chief medical advisor to the Home Office, whom we have encountered regularly in this book.[21] Also present was Dr Edward Mapother, whom Thomas Bewley would later describe as 'the most influential psychiatrist in the first half of the twentieth century', medical director of the Maudsley Hospital and founder of the postgraduate medical school of London University, the precursor of the Institute of Psychiatry.[22] These were joined by Dr Hugh Crichton-Miller, chair of the NCMH subcommittee on the legal restraint of drug addicts, a psychoanalyst and founder of the Tavistock Clinic; by Dr Isabel Wilson, the Committee's only woman member, a leading psychiatrist and senior commissioner to the Board of Control for Lunacy; and by Dr William Norwood East, forensic psychiatrist, medical inspector of H.M. Prisons and inspector of retreats under the Inebriates Acts, whose presence formed an important link with the pre-history of confinement.[23] Dr Walter Russell Brain, a

[18] F. Honigsbaum, *The division in British medicine: a history of the separation of general practice from hospital care, 1911–1968* (New York: St Martin's Press, 1979).

[19] B. Shephard, *A War of Nerves: Soldiers and Psychiatrists in the Twentieth Century 1914–1994* (London: Pimlico, 2000) pp. 163, 181.

[20] J. H. R. Ramsey, 'A King, a Doctor and a Convenient Death' *British Medical Journal*, 308, 6941 (1994) p. 1445.

[21] P. H. A. Willcox, (1970) *Detective Physician: The Life and Work of Sir William Willcox 1870–1941* London: Heinemann.

[22] Thomas Bewley *Madness to Mental Illness. A History of the Royal College of Psychiatrists.* Online archive 13, *Edward Mapother (1881–1940)* http://www.rcpsych.ac.uk/usefulresources/publications/books/rcpp/9781904671350/extra9781904671350.aspx Accessed 15 November 2012.

[23] East, Sir (William) Norwood Oxford Dictionary of National Biography http://www.oxforddnb.com/index/32/101032958/.

highly successful Harley Street consultant and medical author, who would later assume the presidency of the RCP would play a key role; knighted in 1952, Brain chaired the two Interdepartmental Committees on Drug Addiction in 1958–1961 and 1964–1965, the second of which ushered in the 'clinic'-based system of prescribing.[24] Dr R. D. Gillespie, of Guy's Hospital and the University of London, who became chief psychiatrist to the Royal Air Force during the Second World War; and finally the Committee's Secretary Dr Desmond Curran, senior psychiatrist at St George's who would later sit on the Wolfenden Committee. In view of subsequent accounts of the colonisation of addiction treatment by psychiatrists in the 1960s, the extent of psychiatric representation on the Committee in 1938 is notable, as is the presence of multiple links with the monitoring and restriction of socially marginal populations.[25]

Many of these doctors had thriving private practices in the capital's medical district and were consulted by a wealthy and prestigious clientele. Several, such Dawson of Penn, William Willcox and William Norwood East, had close working and advisory relationships with the state. As we saw in Chap. 3, both Dawson of Penn and Willcox had been involved in the celebrity drug case of Brenda Dean Paul, appearing in court as expert witnesses, Penn playing a central role in obtaining her release from court-mandated residential treatment. Their inside knowledge of addiction and its practical location at the interface of medicine and the law must surely have impacted upon the contributions these men made to the work of the RCP Committee.

The Eugenicists Lay Out the Ground

The Committee's terms of reference were: 'To inquire into the problems involved in the treatment of drug addiction and to consider if further legislative powers are necessary for its cure.'[26] At its first meeting in January

[24] Brain, Walter Russell http://www.oxforddnb.com/index/32/101032035/.

[25] For this later infiltration by psychiatrists, see A. S. Trebach, *The Heroin Solution* Second Edition (Bloomington, Indiana: Unlimited Publishing, 2006) pp. 188, 221, *passim*. See also R. Lart, 'Changing Images of the Addict and Addiction: British Medical Perception from Rolleston to Brain' *International Journal on Drug Policy* 3, 3, (1992) pp. 118–125.

[26] MS5911. Royal College of Physicians: Committee on Drug Addiction. Minutes of Meeting, 18 January 1938. The terms of reference originally included alcoholism but were restricted to drug addiction following discussions in which it was judged that the latter would add an unnecessarily controversial dimension to the work.

1938, Dawson of Penn opened the session by elaborating on these terms of reference. He held that they 'introduced a principle of great importance', which involved 'the duty of the medical profession to demonstrate in a practical manner how medical science could contribute to the solution of social problems which were sometimes considered to be outside its scope'.[27] Many offenders against the law were not simple criminals, he said, but instead had 'one foot in crime and one in pathology'.[28] Penn was well known for his eugenics beliefs; one area that has received little attention from historians is his advocacy of addiction, homosexuality and alcoholism as grounds for divorce.[29] Anything that worked to prevent the reproduction of this class of biological misfits he considered supportive of the objectives of eugenics, and suitable for inclusion in British national policy.

Here at the opening session, Penn seized the initiative immediately by placing addiction within a broader space of social deviance upon which the special competences of medicine must be brought to bear. He explained to the meeting that numerous 'unstable individuals' required care and control both for their own good and society's; in contemporary Britain, however, which lacked a proper eugenic grounding for its policies, such people could only be confined if they were either sentenced to prison or could be held under the lunacy laws. Penn argued that the principle of compulsory detention should be widely accepted in Britain and that drug addicts, as relatively uncontroversial cases, would make a convenient strategic target with which to introduce the principle to the political and administrative classes. The wider objective, he believed, was to extend such forms of detention to the entire population of psychopathic and unstable individuals, of which the addict represented a tiny part. Examples of this broader deviant nation comprised both alcoholics and sexual perverts; by the latter term, Penn was referring primarily to homosexuals, whom he had discussed in identical language in other settings: 'homosexuality was a pathological condition .... It had one foot in the realm of disease and was not wholly in the realm of crime'.[30]

According to Penn and the other eugenicists on the Committee, the broader, deviant population of which addicts were a part closely resembled

[27] Royal College of Physicians- Minutes of Meeting, 18 January 1938.

[28] Ibid.

[29] 'Medical Notes in Parliament', British *Medical Journal* 2, 3993 (1937) pp. 144–146.

[30] Quoted in L. A. Hall, *Sex, Gender and Social Change in Britain since 1880* (Basingstoke & London: Macmillan Press, 2000) pp. 144–5.

the category of the ‘social problem group’ proposed by the Board of Control in its 1929 report, which sought to draw attention to individuals who, while not certifiable under the Mental Deficiency Act, were feckless and sexually promiscuous, in addition to being responsible for the majority of crimes. There was a direct parallel between the aims of the Board of Control report and the objectives of the eugenicists on the Committee, who wished to subject to compulsory detention those among ‘the unfit’ who had been convicted of no offence under the law; many were borderline cases, apparently normal, yet who carried within them the germ of vice and degeneracy—they were ‘a race apart’.[31] In both cases, a means of widening the target category had to be devised.

Most of those present at the first meeting were broadly supportive of Dawson of Penn’s argument that medicine had an important social and political role to play in relation to addiction—given that eugenics lay at the intersection of politics and biology, this was to be expected. William Norwood East believed the moment to be ‘opportune for this enquiry, as legislation affecting the criminal laws was to be expected in the near future, proposing amongst other things new forms of preventive detention’.[32]

As well as alluding to the time-honoured public health intervention of segregating groups to counter the infection of the wider society, Norwood East was here referring to the 1938 Criminal Justice Bill, which was introduced by Sir Samuel Hoare and consisted of a number of reform measures which had been subject to longstanding debate, including the abolition of corporal punishment for young offenders.[33] The most apposite aspects of the Bill from the perspective of the RCP Committee were the proposal for courts to include residential elements in probation orders and for forms of detention to be set up. Under the Bill’s provisions, local authorities would receive government grants to establish residential homes for those not covered by the criminal or lunacy laws. There was hope among some members of the Committee that the legislative reforms they sought could be achieved in the context of this Bill.

In summary, then, the first meeting saw the eugenicists gain the high ground. The remainder of the session and the second meeting at the

[31] D. Porter, ‘Eugenics and the Sterilisation Debate in Sweden and Britain before World War Two’ *Scandinavian Journal of History* 24, 2 (1999) pp. 145–162.

[32] Royal College of Physicians. Minutes of Meeting 18 January 1938.

[33] The 1938 Criminal Justice Bill is discussed in W. Norwood East, ‘The Problem of Alcohol and Drug Addiction in Relation to Crime’, *British Journal of Inebriety* 37,2 (1939) pp. 55–73.

beginning of February were spent in drawing an outline of the inquiry's proposed work in the light of Penn's eugenic principles. In addition, it was agreed that members would concentrate on addiction to five drugs: morphine, heroin, cocaine, opium and its derivatives and, at the urging of Norwood East who claimed that the police would find its inclusion useful, Indian hemp. As we saw in Chap. 4, the use of Indian hemp had apparently expanded in the West End of London during the late 1930s. Finally, it was decided that the Committee would seek the advice of Major William H. Coles, then chief inspector of the Home Office Drugs Branch, in relation to the current dimensions of drug use in Britain. In the event, there was comparatively little focus on Indian hemp in discussions that emerged out of the subsequent meetings.

The British System and the Principle of Compulsion: Interview with Major Coles

The discussion with Major Coles took place on February 22, 1938, and addressed the dimensions and composition of the addict population as currently known to the Home Office. According to Coles, the total was at this point made up of some 630 individuals, of which 305 were men and 325 women. Of this sum, 145 were members of the medical profession—135 men and 10 women. He explained the processes by which addicts became identified by the authorities, the accuracy of the data and the arguments for and against compulsory notification by doctors.[34]

Much of Coles' contribution consisted in an account of the 'nuts and bolts' functioning of the British System. It included the issue of 'medical mismanagement' as an initiator of addiction, Coles hinting that some doctors showed insufficient caution in supplying pain relief in their therapeutic practice. However, this led on to the key themes of the interview, which clustered around the effectiveness or otherwise of current treatment methods, and the respective strengths of voluntary and compulsory detention. Professor Mapother responded that the Maudsley was presently unwilling to admit drug addicts at all, the available modes of treatment being in his view so unsatisfactory. Most addicts would not subject themselves voluntarily to a cure, he claimed, and, if they did so, discharged themselves too soon to achieve any lasting abstinence. The Committee

[34] RCP Committee on Drug Addiction: Report on Discussion with Major E.H. Coles of the Home Office on 22nd February 1938.

agreed that voluntary treatment was generally ineffective, since addicts were unwilling to remain in detention for sufficient length of time. Consequently, 'it would be desirable to have power to detain a drug addict because he was a drug addict and for no other reason'.[35] The element of compulsion, broadly absent from the present arrangements, was, declared Mapother, essential if successful outcomes were to be achieved.

Coles explained to the meeting that any such proposals radically departed from the existing legislation; he showed considerable caution when asked whether this type of move would meet with approval at the Home Office. As the minutes record, he 'found himself unable to express an opinion as to how such a proposal for change in the legal position would be greeted in official circles'.[36] It is notable that Coles was, on this issue, at odds with Sir William Willcox, who had repeatedly indicated that the Home Office would welcome legislative change in order to permit stricter controls to be exercised over addicts. Willcox reiterated this point several times across the series of meetings. Coles, by contrast, retained in general a reserved stance in relation to the Committee's questioning, adding only that, in order to be effective, detention would require not just sufficient time in which to secure withdrawal but a further period to allow for rehabilitation and aftercare.

Significantly, the sole occasion on which Coles prompted the membership to adopt a measure came when the discussions touched on the problem of overprescribing doctors supplying nonmedical or vicious addicts. Asked about this population by the Committee, Coles expressed his opinion that, since there was no organised traffic, it was doctors who constituted the source of illicit drugs in the UK. He suggested the possibility of setting up a panel of doctors to whom practitioners would be required to refer cases before they were allowed to prescribe narcotics and explained the present procedures by which doctors could be required to submit to an undertaking in relation to their drug prescribing. Coles then reminded the Committee that the Home Secretary was able to withdraw a practitioner's authority to prescribe only after they had been convicted of an offence under the dangerous drugs laws. He wondered aloud whether the Committee judged it preferable if the Home Secretary was to be given the power to withdraw a doctor's authority 'in proper cases' *prior* to any offence being committed. Such an intervention in relation to doctors was

[35] Ibid.
[36] Ibid.

in stark contrast to Norwood East's cautious statements with respect to compulsory measures for addicts.

Coles next raised the topic of the tribunals that had been included in the recommendations of the Rolleston Committee and had been designed precisely in order to deal with overprescribing doctors. However, he described the tribunal—which had yet to be utilised—as something that was 'cumbersome and would involve great publicity'; he invited the RCP Committee to devise some other, more effective measure.[37]

This was a somewhat curious stance, since these tribunals offered a ready-made method of dealing with the problems he had just identified. Nonetheless, the hostility on the part of the Home Office toward the medical tribunals described in the Rolleston Report was of long standing. It has been remarked upon by Spear but has never been adequately accounted for.[38] Coles' remarks before the RCP Committee indicate that it was engendered partly because of the 'cumbersome' mechanisms involved, which suffered from the disadvantages of the criminal justice system, and partly because of the publicity it entailed. In addition, one can speculate that the Home Office may have been reluctant to make use of the medical tribunal while there appeared to be the possibility of some other method which was both more streamlined and more discreet: a method whereby the Home Secretary could exercise his power to withdraw the authority to prescribe from a given practitioner without the need for any intervention by the courts. Given his hints and suggestions, it appears that Coles was hoping the RCP Committee might suggest some suitable mechanism along these lines. On a more general note, his interventions around this point make it clear that, while the Home Office was often relatively comfortable with the existence of a small population of addicts, it was prepared to be much more proactive in its pursuit of lax prescribers—the script doctors, 'broken-down medical men' and their ilk, whom it viewed as sources of a particularly contagious mode of addiction.

The session with Major Coles has been examined in some detail in order to provide an understanding of both the content and the tone of proceedings and of the position of the Home Office in relation to the Committee's early proposals. It was apparent that the Committee was moving strongly in favour of reconfiguring the British System along much

[37] Ibid.

[38] H. B. Spear, *Heroin Addiction, Care and Control*, pp. 45–46.

more stringent lines; the Home Office, meanwhile, had been restrained in its responses, except with regard to those doctors prescribing for addicts, whose conduct it clearly saw as lying at the heart of the problem of contemporary British addiction, and in relation to whom it was prepared to contemplate stricter measures.

The Eugenicists' Attempt to Consolidate

The subsequent meeting in late March reviewed the themes prominent in the discussion with Coles, and a number of points were agreed by the Committee, the most important of which for our purposes were as follows:

that the present facilities for treating addiction were 'inadequate and unsatisfactory';
that the setting up of effective treatment would require changes in the law;
that, if practicable, legislation was also desirable in order to establish compulsory treatment and to protect the property and family of the addict;
that compulsory detention should include a period of withdrawal supplemented by a period of rehabilitation;
that the detoxification period should not exceed three months and that a further period of up to two years would be appended, as necessary;
that there would be a follow-up phase during which the addict would be reviewed for signs of drug use;
and that the use of drugs during this period should constitute a criminal offence.

While Penn was unable to attend this meeting, he telephoned his comments regarding the discussion with Coles, and returned to the broader themes he had invoked in his introductory remarks. 'It is not only a question of dope', he insisted.[39] He was strongly in favour of compulsion, which 'might include a revival of the old term of "preventive detention", i.e. detaining people for the purpose of treatment which would be compulsory ... such detention might be a way of treating certain sexual offences as well as drug addicts ...'.[40] Penn's case rested on the judgement that, 'There is no way of treating a great many of the cases of drug addic-

[39] Royal College of Physicians—Telephone message from Lord Dawson of Penn 21.3.38.
[40] Ibid.

tion except by compulsory detention'.[41] Compulsion, he concluded, was 'a feature of legislation to which we must convert our legal authorities'.[42]

Confining the Deviant Nation: Tactical Disparities

At the fifth session in June, Dawson of Penn once more pressed his case for the principle of compulsion to be applied to the entire deviant nation. He argued that the real importance of addiction, a numerically tiny problem in British society, lay in its representation of much more widespread social deviance. What was required was an institution in which all these marginal subjectivities might be assembled for treatment and cure. While some would be detained upon conviction, Penn believed it was essential that others be incarcerated 'before they had actually committed any crime or antisocial act'.[43] Drug addicts, for example, should be committed on grounds of their addiction per se. Some technical discussion ensued as to the precise mechanisms that might be employed to achieve this objective.

The Chairman then raised the tactical question that was to divide the Committee for the remainder of its existence—namely, 'whether definite recommendations should be made with regard to the treatment of drug addiction as a separate problem, or whether it should be said that such treatment would only be practicable and desirable as part of a larger problem'.[44] On this point the Committee as a whole is minuted as agreeing with the general terms of Penn's thought: compulsion was both essential for addicts and best understood as applicable to the deviant nation as a whole. Here Willcox interjected to restate his belief that the Home Office would welcome measures specific to addicts; however, he felt that the larger problem might be considered 'more fruitfully' at a later date. Mapother countered by expressing the opinion that, were legislation to be secured to deal with addiction alone, it would be a disappointing result, as the prognosis for the treatment of addicts was so poor that it would be liable to ruin the prospect for broader reforms. Unsurprisingly, Penn repeated his view that any report for which the Committee was responsible must emphasise the broader deviant context of which addiction was a part.

[41] Ibid.
[42] Ibid.
[43] Royal College of Physicians- Minutes of Meeting 9th June 1938.
[44] Ibid.

With disparate positions being voiced on the question of tactics, the Chairman proposed that, prior to the next meeting, he would issue a questionnaire on which members might give their views on some of the practical issues still to be settled. The meeting closed with an apparent consensus having been achieved but with the first signs of disagreement hovering at the margins.

Dissent on the Committee: Russell Brain and the Minority Report

The disagreement regarding strategy, which had over the months been percolating quietly, now began to surface. The Chairman moved that the Committee should agree that addiction must be dealt with not as an isolated question but as part of a larger problem. Penn was quick to assent. Crichton-Miller, meanwhile, intervened pragmatically to state that he was in favour of 'the method that would bring the greatest practical results in the shortest space of time' and while wishing in principle to deal with the larger problem, he was concerned that such a course could result in delays and postponement for the addiction issue.[45] Russell Brain, who was a Quaker and well known for his reticence, had until this juncture made relatively little contribution to the deliberations; now, however, he spoke up forcefully, emerging as the Committee's leading dissenter.[46] While himself a member of the Eugenics Society, Brain's approach was considerably more pragmatic than that of his antagonists and less wedded to eugenicist ideology. First, he argued that it would be very difficult to define the large and heterogeneous problem of psychopathology; addiction to drugs was, by contrast, a small and well-delineated domain; by attempting to capture the broader issue, they risked 'losing the substance in pursuit of the Shadow'[47] and miring the entire project in controversy. Those who sought to incarcerate the deviant nation made their disagreement known.

The July meeting was not followed by another until November. In the interim, the differences flared up into a full-blown dispute. Brain had written to Secretary Curran in July, commenting archly that, 'I can hardly bear to think of the "Talk Addiction Committee" spending another two years

[45] Ibid.

[46] G. Pickering, 'Brain, Walter Russell, first Baron Brain (1895–1966)', rev. *Oxford Dictionary of National Biography*, (Oxford: Oxford University Press, 2004), http://www.oxforddnb.com/index/32/101032035/Accessed 07.10 2013.

[47] Royal College of Physicians- Minutes of Meeting, 4 July 1938.

discussing what should be done with the psychopathic.'[48] Remarks such as this suggest that, despite his public reserve, Brain had been exasperated by the discussions, and regarded his own position as a pragmatic one constructed in contrast to the ideological proposals expounded by Penn and Mapother. Writing to Curran and to Chairman Bernard Hart, he enclosed a statement of his views, which he believed 'will be opposed to the Report you are now drafting, and if so I would like them appended as a minority report'.[49] Brain claimed that there was more support for his opinions amongst the Committee than might have been apparent at the July meeting, and argued that 'the future plans of the Committee are extremely vague, and that whereas agreement could probably be obtained for administrative measures with regard to drug addicts, an attempt at the moment to include the miscellaneous group of psychopathic individuals is likely to lead only to controversy'.[50] He concluded by adding that he was in possession of 'private information that the Home Office (was) very sceptical of the value of psychological treatment for the group of individuals, whom Dawson characterises as having one foot in crime and one foot in pathology'.[51] The source of this private information was not disclosed.

Brain's memorandum referred to that well-defined group of addicts whose condition could be diagnosed with certainty and whose treatment was generally agreed; moreover, he said, it was widely felt that a degree of compulsion was appropriate in these cases. He contrasted addicts to the

> larger group of psychopathic individuals in general, which includes alcohol addicts and the sexually abnormal. These persons ... are much more difficult to define, and there is far less agreement as to what is the appropriate treatment, and it is difficult to say which, if any, require to be deprived of their liberty for therapeutic as distinct from punitive purposes.[52]

Brain therefore argued that it would be a mistake to postpone the attempt to solve the relatively minor problem until they could devise a solution to the larger one; instead, the 'wiser practical course is to press for measures for the treatment of drug addicts now'.[53] Such a strategy, moreover, would 'obtain recognition for a principle, namely compulsory treat-

[48] RCP Committee 1938- Brain to Curran, 16 July 1938.
[49] RCP Committee 1938- Brain to Hart, 18 July 1938.
[50] Ibid.
[51] Ibid.
[52] RCP Committee 1938- Memorandum from Russell Brain.
[53] Ibid.

ment of persons not of unsound mind, the application of which might later be extended'.[54]

The Chair's Attempts at Compromise

The Committee's November meeting took place without Dawson of Penn and centred on a memorandum circulated by the Chairman. The document summarised the present position of the Committee's deliberations, acknowledging that while the July meeting had passed the resolution to treat addiction as a component of a broader problem, it did so with considerable reluctance and that Russell Brain and Crichton-Miller had subsequently written to the Chairman elaborating a dissenting view and requesting that it be appended as a minority report. Meanwhile, Mapother had submitted written opinion in the course of responding to the questionnaire and was wholly committed to the majority position. After studying the conflicting arguments, Hart judged that 'no compromise between the two standpoints would seem to be possible'.[55] In such an impasse, he told them, his duty as chair was to try to find some way forward, and he began by offering two potential courses. The first, he explained, was to submit the report as it had been proposed at the July meeting, appending the views of Russell Brain as a minority report; the second would involve the submission of a report outlining the agreed views of the Committee regarding the need for legislative reform to permit compulsory treatment of addicts, and a statement that addiction, along with alcoholism and sex perversions, formed part of a larger problem requiring a combination of legal and therapeutic measures, but that there was no agreement amongst members either to seek measures dealing with addicts alone or to concentrate on the broader deviant population. The problem with these weakened positions was, according to Hart, that 'a Report along either of these lines would be unlikely to eventuate in any action being taken by the Comitia, or ultimately by the Legislature'.[56] Whichever course was taken, he believed there should be an emphasis on the need to control the addict's property and affairs, and he anticipated general agreement on this point.

The same divisions marked the Committee's discussions at its November session. Gillespie began by contending that legislation dealing with addicts

[54] Ibid.

[55] RCP Committee 1938- Chairman's Memorandum 2, October 1938.

[56] Ibid.

alone would be neither feasible nor expedient, and the terms of reference should be expanded to cover the full psychopathic population. Brain, for his part, was eager to stress that the dispute was an administrative one rather than a medical disagreement: it was a question of what was practical. The small size of the addict population need not present a hindrance; after all, he noted correctly, the group was already the object of 'a mass of legislation dealing with drugs'.[57] Curran informed members that he had heard the undersecretary of state express the view that public opinion would not tolerate the compulsory detention of alcoholics. It was agreed that the Committee would invite Sir Oscar Dowson, legal advisor to the Home Office, to attend the next meeting along with Major Coles with a view to obtaining expert opinion as to the practicality of the Committee's proposals. Isabel Wilson agreed to consult Sir Hubert Bond, commissioner at the Board of Control for Lunacy and Mental Deficiency until his death in 1945, on the question of whether Section 116 of the Lunacy Act would permit compulsory detention. In the event, Bernard Hart interviewed Sir Claude Schuster, permanent secretary to the Lord Chancellor, on the question, but was unable to make much headway. Schuster promised to make further inquiries and to acquaint the Chairman with their results. By that time, however, the Committee's work had fallen victim to the institutional inertia accompanying the approach of the Second World War.

The RCP Committee on Drug Addiction: Another Failure for Eugenics

The discussion with Dowson and Coles took place prior to the final Committee meeting on December 7, 1938. It commenced with Hart asking his two experts, 'Was it likely that the proposed legislation would be contemplated, or would be practical, in order to deal with the problem of drug addiction?'[58] Hart reminded them of the Committee's views in relation to the need for legislative change and the introduction of a new principle of compulsory detention that would apply to individuals who were neither criminal nor insane. Dowson responded by stating that any move to restrict the liberty of the subject aroused opposition, and required,

[57] RCP Committee 1938- Minutes of Meeting, 9 November 1938.

[58] RCP Committee 1938- Report of discussion with Sir Oscar Dowson and Major Coles, 7 December 1938.

therefore, the support of a very strong case prior to any discussion in parliament. Given the dimensions of the drug addict population, he found it hard to envisage parliament making such changes in the law. Consequently, he believed that the prospect of achieving the Committee's objectives in this field was 'very remote'.[59] He wondered whether the argument could be made that drug addicts constituted a 'social menace'. Such a status represented perhaps the only chance of achieving it. At this point, Major Coles interjected with the opinion that, again in view of their small numbers, it was most unlikely that drug addicts would be classified in this way.[60]

Crichton-Miller asked a question that he had raised previously, namely, whether (as claimed by Willcox) the Home Office would 'welcome fresh legislation for drug addicts'.[61] Coles replied that the issue had never received official consideration. He continued: 'Those who had to deal with drug addicts would welcome legislation which would enable them to deal more effectively with the problem.'[62] He added, however, an important qualification: '…but they appreciated that it would not be possible to approach parliament for far reaching powers in order to deal with such a very small group'.[63] The question of making addiction per se a crime was also raised, but Coles was similarly sceptical in this regard, his argument hinging on the difference between drug addicts and alcoholics, with the former generally only manifesting a 'gross impairment of efficiency' when deprived of drugs.[64] This was, he said, in contrast to the typical 'drunk and disorderly', whose condition worsened when supplied with alcohol. Asked whether the principle of compulsory detention could be extended to the larger group of psychopathic individuals, Dowson replied that the same considerations of the liberty of the subject applied to this larger population and feared that the task of defining the psychopathic would prove 'baffling'.[65] He foresaw endless disagreements between doctors regarding who was and was not a psychopath. Professor Mapother countered that the problem of definition was 'theoretical rather than real'.[66] There was no

[59] Dowson, in Ibid.
[60] Coles, in Ibid.
[61] Crichton-Miller in Ibid.
[62] Coles in Ibid.
[63] Ibid.
[64] Ibid.
[65] Dowson in Ibid.
[66] Mapother in Ibid.

accepted definition of insanity, he said, but despite this it was possible to certify an individual, and he believed that in practice the identification of addiction would be substantially agreed.

Penn made reference to the Children's Acts, arguing that they and the Criminal Justice Bill now going through parliament 'reflected the increasing demand by modern opinion of the necessity for the treatment of certain offenders'.[67] Just as the Bill recommended detention for certain delinquents, the Committee sought to extend the principle to include 'the preventive detention and treatment of such persons as drug addicts and sexual perverts who were potentially antisocial, although they might not have committed any crime'.[68] Dowson responded that the only way those who had committed no crime could be included under the Bill's provisions was if their condition itself were to become an offence. There was some debate as to whether a law to deal with addiction could be introduced along the lines of the Lunacy Acts; at this point, Mapother advocated the formation of a new body analogous to the Children's Court, featuring both medically trained and lay members, before which a psychopathic individual could be brought by a doctor or the police. Dowson was once again doubtful about the suggestion, judging that 'such a proposal would be completely outside the scope of the Criminal Justice Bill'.[69]

Following their abortive interview with Dowson and Coles, the Committee members met for the final time. They decided that, in the light of the advice received from the Home Office experts, 'it would be undesirable to make any recommendation to deal with Drug Addiction per se, and that they should present an interim report to the January Comitia asking that the terms of reference of the Committee should be extended'.[70] In the event, no final report was produced, Hart and Curran instead authoring a three-page 'Summary of Position' providing an overview of the conclusions reached by the Committee. This document did its best to present a patina of unanimity, but given the disagreements structuring the debates, it remained an ambivalent text. The Committee had agreed that 'the present facilities for the treatment of drug addiction ... are inadequate and unsatisfactory ...'.[71] Effective treatment, it continued, would require

[67] Penn in Ibid.

[68] Ibid.

[69] Dowson in Ibid.

[70] Royal College of Physicians Committee 1938- Minutes of Meeting 7 December 1938.

[71] Royal College of Physicians Committee 1938- Summary of the position reached by the Committee on Drug Addiction.

legislative change, and it was desirable to establish compulsory treatment and to protect the addict's family and property. As addiction to drugs was so limited in Britain, it was doubtful that the legislature would make such changes, which involved the introduction of a new legal principle—namely, the detention of individuals who were neither criminal nor insane. Moreover, the document claimed, the country's existing treatment facilities were inadequate to the task, while the establishment of new ones was unlikely due to the size of the addict population. Following the opinion of Mapother, it commented that the results of the current treatment of addicts were disappointing.

The divisions on the Committee were then acknowledged. Some members believed that addiction could not and should not be dealt with in isolation from the broader family of social deviants, such as alcoholics and sexual perverts. While there was agreement that this wider class would benefit from compulsory treatment, some felt that the establishment of such treatment was probably not a practical measure. Accordingly, the issue facing the Committee was that the small numbers of addicts in practice prevented the achievement of the reforms that the members judged to be necessary; at the same time, if the terms of reference were extended to embrace the wider deviant nation, a larger population would be constituted, but there would be new problems, such as that of arriving at a legally acceptable definition. In conclusion, the document stated that: 'The Committee felt that the time had come to seek advice and guidance as to what might be feasible from the administrative point of view as regards the larger problem of the "psychopath".'[72]

With the approach of war in 1939, the movement toward compulsory detention faded from public view and political priority. The Committee, divided in its objectives, was unable to inject sufficient impetus into its project to propel it into the policy realm. This was mainly the result of the intervention of Russell Brain and Crichton-Miller, since the remainder of members seemed willing to support the proposals emanating from Dawson of Penn and Mapother. It is notable too that the Home Office, which has sometimes been identified as the repository of a repressive disciplinary perspective with regard to addicts, gave little in the way of encouragement to those seeking to modify the law to permit the detention of individuals who were classified as neither sick nor criminal. Had the Committee been less ambitious in scope and limited its objectives to dealing with drug

[72] Ibid.

addicts instead of attempting to confine a large and amorphous population, it may have enjoyed more encouragement from the Home Office. Had its proposals been translated into policy, the face of the classic British System would have been radically altered, with maintenance doses of drugs being replaced by a preventive medico-penal confinement that could sequester individuals for approximately three years, with a follow-up period during which abstinence was monitored and any return to drug use criminalised. In a sense, what was advocated by Penn and his faction was a final attempt to respond to addiction in terms of a disciplinary framework, with segregation and confinement at its heart. It was a programme that belonged to the nineteenth century. What would take its place in later decades would be much more in line with the technocratic ethic that characterised Russell Brain's interventions, with addicts remaining in the community, and it was Brain that steered the 1964–1965 Interdepartmental Committee that put the new arrangements into place.

The Criminal Justice Act of 1948 and the Postwar Re-emergence of Compulsion

Despite the inertia that overcame its work at the close of a year's discussion—no report was made—many of the themes that had dominated the RCP Committee on Drug Addiction surfaced again in the immediate aftermath of the Second World War. Moreover, this time it was the Home Office that provided the driving force. The context was once again the passage through parliament of the modified Criminal Justice Bill, which was drafted in 1947 and passed the following year; again, there were discussions as to whether the Bill might provide a lawful means of detaining addicts. The call came from the Lord Chancellor.

In March 1947, Coles wrote to Sir Wilson Jameson, chief medical officer at the Ministry of Health and former dean of the London School of Hygiene and Tropical Medicine, informing him that the Home Office was again giving special consideration to 'the problem of the control and cure of drug addicts' and asking for a medical officer from the Ministry to attend a 'small, informal' meeting to be held the following week.[73] Coles enclosed an outline of the proposed discussion and included an excerpt from a letter sent by William Jowett, Lord Chancellor, to the Home Secretary. It contained a paragraph in which Jowett declared that he

[73] TNA MH 135/157, Letter from Coles to Jameson, 14 March 1947.

'would like to see some home to which … drug fiends could be sent from which they would not be able to escape and at which they could receive appropriate treatment. I would like it to be as little like a prison as possible: much more like a nursing home, but the one essential is that they should stay there until they are cured'.[74]This letter was inspired by a story featured in the national press in February, which the Lord Chancellor had read. It dealt with the case of two Mayfair women prosecuted for the possession of heroin. Maureen Brazil and Cynthia Force, 'two smartly dressed women', were allowed bail on the understanding that they would enter a nursing home to undergo addiction treatment.[75] 'What a God-send it would be for those two unhappy girls we are reading about in the papers today if they could be sent to such a place and there kept under medical observation until this craving for heroin had gone', commented the Lord Chancellor, illustrating once more the extent to which newspaper reporting of drug court cases extended not only to the general public but to highly placed policy-makers.[76]

Coles' preparatory notes for the meeting, which would be chaired by himself and attended by Frank Thornton and representatives from the Prisons Commission and the Board of Control, began with a critical discussion of the present system. 'As the law stands', he explained, 'it is *not* an offence to be a drug addict.'[77] There were three groups that were particularly problematic on account of the shape of British legislation: those who used preparations containing less than 0.2 per cent of morphine, which could be legally obtained from pharmacies; addict doctors who prescribed drugs for themselves; and finally, 'the irresponsible group including prostitutes and their male associates who obtain supplies *lawfully* on the prescriptions of certain doctors'.[78] The linkage made here between drug addiction and the commercial sex trade gives an indication of a theme which will be increasingly important in the 1950s, as London sought to remove prostitutes and homosexuals from the flagrant visibility of the streets.[79] At the subsequent meeting, it was stated that of 350 known

[74] TNA MH 135/157, Extract from letter from Lord Chancellor to Home Secretary, 18 February 1947.

[75] *Daily Mirror*, 21 February 1947, p. 3.

[76] Ibid.

[77] TNA MH 135/157, 'Notes on the Control and Cure of Drug Addicts' (emphasis original).

[78] Ibid. (emphasis original).

[79] Mort, *Capital Affairs*, pp. 139–196, *passim*.

addicts, there were 'only about 100 vicious addicts against whom proceedings might be taken'.[80] It was further pointed out in Coles' memorandum that, with an estimated 75,000 doctors on the register and 350 known addicts, most were likely to have little or no experience of dealing with addiction. Doctors implicated in the supply of drugs are given slightly more detailed consideration by breaking them down into three categories: script doctors, here defined by Coles in the following terms: 'These men issue prescriptions at high fees with little regard to the needs of the case and the prospect of cure', while 'weak but well-meaning doctors' and 'self-styled experts' are classified separately.[81]

The dominant concern of this meeting lay for the Home Office in finding solutions to the problems of control it had identified in its preparatory memorandum, which discussed the possibility of providing state nursing homes to which addicts could be compulsorily consigned. According to Coles, in the first instance, a lack of government funds had stymied the proposals of the 1938 RCP Committee. Coles' second suggestion was to 'establish control', apparently dealing now with the policing side of the divide implicit in the Home Office concept of 'cure and control'. As the document states: 'The best course here would seem to be the making of addiction per se an offence with power of committal to a state institution.'[82] It proposed three years in such a facility as 'a reasonable time for the re-education of the addict', with general oversight residing in the Drugs Branch.[83]

Other themes examined at length by the RCP Committee were now discussed at the Home Office, including the problems of legally defining addiction and the type of institutions required. In practical policy terms, the discussions produced three suggestions: firstly, await the re-writing of the Lunacy and Mental Treatment Acts (then under consideration), and make addiction a reason for certification; secondly, devise a scheme along the lines of the power of committal to an approved institution under the Public Health Act, as was done for those TB patients considered to represent a public health hazard; and finally, as Coles had indicated in his notes as a preferred option, render addiction itself a criminal offence. It was argued that the best location for the confinement of addicts would be 'the new clinic for psychopaths' currently envisaged by the Prisons Commission.[84]

[80] TNA MH 135/157, 'Meeting at Home Office, 1 April 1947'.
[81] TNA MH 135/157, 'Notes on the Control and Cure of Drug Addicts'.
[82] Ibid.
[83] Ibid.
[84] TNA MH 135/157, 'Meeting at Home Office, 1 April 1947'.

The Home Office's meeting of April 1947 resurrected the major themes of the RCP Committee on Drug Addiction, though it is notable that the discussions steered well away from the question of the deviant population in general, a theme that belonged to the eugenic adventure which had probably prevented the Committee's deliberations from progressing to the level of policy-making. Like eugenic interventions more generally, it failed in its objective of inspiring the legislation necessary to implement its programme. Except for the tentative proposal that addicts could be treated in an as-yet inbuilt clinic for psychopaths, the 1947 meeting remained focused firmly on addiction, which perhaps gives us a further intimation that the lukewarm support shown by Coles for the RCP Committee's project resulted from the department's wariness toward the grand gestures of Penn and Mapother. Nevertheless, it provides further evidence of discontent with the classical British System, this time amongst the senior figures at the Home Office who were entrusted with its oversight. Once again it is likely that the parlous condition of the British economy after six years of ruinous war against the Axis powers left the state lacking sufficient funds to act upon the advice of its experts. The regulatory architecture was to remain intact through the years of austerity. By the time major changes came to be wrought in the 1960s, the size of the British addict population had expanded significantly, and a range of different forms of drug use had taken hold amongst the new youth culture; the changed conditions resulted in a different regime from that envisaged by either the Royal College of Physicians Committee on Drug Addiction or the Home Office of Coles and Thornton.

CHAPTER 7

Morphine and Morale: The British System and the Second World War

Introduction

While this chapter retains the focus of the previous on medical opinion and practice with respect to addiction, it deals primarily with the problems arising from regulating morphine under emergency conditions on the Second World War Home Front, which posed a somewhat different type of challenge for the British System. Despite its often being understood as purely a system of prohibition, the crux of twentieth-century drug control lay in balancing the enabling role of the state with regard to drugs—which involved ensuring the availability of adequate supplies to meet medical and scientific needs—with its restrictive function, which sought to deny access to those same drugs for nonmedical purposes such as entertainment and pleasure.

This chapter illustrates both dimensions of drug control at work; in the Second World War, the UK Home Front posed this problem of balance to the government in a particularly acute and immediate way. In order to meet the medical requirements that were anticipated to arise from mass bombing of cities from the air—in terms of both bodily wounds and mass panic—stocks of morphine came to be spread much more densely throughout the population than they were under peacetime conditions. The state was required by war to ensure that access to pain relief was available to both the armed forces and the civilian population.

Simultaneously, in the chaos and carnage of a total war in which the entire population was expected to play its part, it would prove doubly

C. Hallam, *White Drug Cultures and Regulation in London, 1916–1960*, https://doi.org/10.1007/978-3-319-94770-9_7

difficult to limit the access of these powerful analgesics to the medical practitioners who were exclusively authorised to prescribe and administer them. Broadly speaking, in what became a wartime struggle between two state institutions, the Ministry of Health embodied the enabling function with respect to drugs, while the Home Office played the role of restriction. It was a tricky balance, for the customary attempts by the authorities to suppress nonmedical forms of drug taking had to be carried on throughout the conflict if Britain was to meet its international treaty obligations.

Drugs and World War

The First World War injected a dynamic force into the control regime, which had been crystallising through the process leading to the International Opium Convention, agreed at The Hague in 1912 (The Hague Convention). While considerable disparity of views remained amongst the participating nations, these were neatly resolved via the incorporation of The Hague Convention into the Versailles peace treaty in 1919. Crucially, this meant that two of what were seen as the most recalcitrant of the drug-producing nations, Germany and Turkey, were compelled to adopt restrictive measures in order to bring hostilities to an end. As diplomatic historian William McAllister observes: 'With the stroke of a pen, the requirement of the 1912 treaty for near-universal adherence was satisfied.'[1] The ratification of The Hague Convention required signatory states to enact domestic legislation along the lines elaborated in the treaty, with a range of drugs to be limited to 'medical and legitimate' purposes.[2] While Britain's 1920 Dangerous Drugs Act represented the fulfilment of its Hague treaty obligations, another legal instrument preceded the act and was driven directly by wartime circumstances. This was section 40b of the DORA, which in 1916 deployed emergency legislation to restrict the possession and trafficking of opium and cocaine. According to Virginia Berridge, the move was prompted primarily by anxieties regarding the alleged rapid spread of cocaine use by soldiers on leave in the West End of London, and by the smuggling of opium and morphine to the Far East on board British vessels.[3] The legislation was superseded by the 1920

[1] McAllister, *Drug Diplomacy*, p. 37.

[2] The International Opium Convention, article IX, in The *American Journal of International Law*, 6,3, Supplement: Official Documents, (1912), pp. 177–192.

[3] Berridge, 'War Conditions and Narcotics Control'.

Dangerous Drugs Act, and the First World War is therefore rightly seen as a key turning point in the initiation of the international control regime, which bore directly on national legislation.

The Second World War meanwhile led to the demise of the old League of Nations-administered system, giving way to a regime in which the USA was unambiguously the directing force in drug control arrangements reconfigured under the auspices of the newly inaugurated United Nations. The USA pushed for reform along more restrictive lines, and, eventually, the Single Convention on Narcotic Drugs of 1961 replaced a complex set of international and bilateral instruments as the legal foundation for control, and endures in this role to the present.[4,5] The war also impacted powerfully upon the locations of production and routes of supply of illicit drugs, with the secret service arms of several states entering into covert relationships with organised criminal groups.[6] These often extended tacit licence to traffickers to operate their businesses, within certain limits, in exchange for intelligence and other expertise that only the traffickers possessed.

The Regulatory Background: The Home Office Drugs Branch at War

In the late 1930s, Britain contemplated the approach of the Second World War and with it the threat of massive air raids that would not only cause bodily wounds and injuries but also constitute a profound threat to the morale of the population on the Home Front.[7] Elements in the medical profession and the government believed that it would be essential to have plentiful and widespread stocks of morphine ready to hand in order to deal

[4] The Single Convention was followed by the two further UN conventions that together form the basis of the global system, Convention on Psychotropic Substances, 1971 and the United Nations Convention Against Illicit Traffic in Narcotic Drugs and Psychoptropic Substances, 1988.

[5] Though the system may be coming under unprecedented pressure to change due to a complex set of recent developments. See D. R. Bewley-Taylor, *International Drug Control: Consensus Fractured*. Cambridge: Cambridge University Press, (2012). See also D. R. Bewley-Taylor, & M. Jelsma, (2012) Regime Change: Revisiting the 1961 Single Convention on Narcotic Drugs *International Journal of Drug Policy* 23,1 (2012) pp. 72–81.

[6] A. W. McCoy, (2003) *The Politics of Heroin: CIA Complicity in the Global Drugs Trade* (Chicago: Lawrence Hill, 2003) and P. A. Chouvy, *Opium: Uncovering the Politics of the Poppy* (London: I.B. Taurus, 2009).

[7] S. R. Grayzel, *At Home and Under Fire: Air Raids and Culture in Britain from the Great War to the Blitz* (Cambridge: Cambridge University Press, 2012).

with these eventualities. Contemporary debates focused on the regulation of supplies in three main contexts, though in practice these would overlap in multiple ways. The first and most important setting related to the storage and use of morphine at First Aid Posts and the Mobile Units that were attached to them, in circumstances where no doctor was present to address the immediate needs of casualties; secondly, the availability of morphine in invasion conditions, especially in remote rural areas or potential landing zones when no doctor was likely to be available (and the related question of whether to allow District Nurses to access and administer morphine); finally, the siting of and access to supplies at specific locations where casualties were anticipated—for example, tube stations functioning as public air raid shelters. In each of these spaces, the problem was essentially the same: how to manage the expanded supply of morphine, and whether legislative and regulatory changes would prove necessary to increase flexibility and ensure that citizens would receive adequate pain relief, which was the medical contention, or, in order to protect the public from the ever-present threat of addiction, the existing tight restrictions should remain intact, which was the Home Office position.[8] In the event, after spending many months in a largely fruitless attempt to confine control of morphine to the hands of doctors, the Home Office would find itself shifting toward a pragmatism which, while it avoided legislative changes, turned a blind eye to the irregular use of morphine in a variety of wartime settings.

The provision of morphine within these contexts had been factored into the calculation of national morale, and numerous medical practitioners, who were schooled throughout the 1930s in the theory that the heavy bombing of cities was liable to generate mass hysteria among citizens, argued that a greater flexibility would be essential to meet the expanded need for morphine. According to the regulations obtaining under the Dangerous Drugs Act, only medical practitioners were authorised to supply morphine, and only then to individuals in possession of a legitimate prescription. However, it was argued by various officials at the Ministry of Health and by many doctors that in wartime conditions these requirements would have to be relaxed in order to satisfy medical need.

[8] HO 45/21172 'Relaxation of regulations to allow administration of morphine by approved persons in war emergency conditions. Control and storage of drugs at wartime first aid posts and in factories under government administration.' (1938–1947); MH 76/83 'Equipment; storage of dangerous drugs 1939–1945.'

The contention was that Air Raid Precautions (ARP) workers, nurses and various others engaged in the provision of frontline civil defence services should be enabled to administer morphine if the circumstances so demanded.

The necessity of making morphine supplies more readily available to the general population in case of emergency confronted the British regulatory system with a major wartime challenge and was the period's most significant issue for the country's drugs-related governance. It found the Home Office attempting to reconcile and balance the imperative of greater access to drugs against the impulse toward restriction that had guided drug policy since the First World War. In the words of Frank Thornton, who had joined the Home Office Drugs Branch in 1917 during its formative years, while the medical profession was sovereign over the administration of drugs to patients, the Branch's main concern:

> is in safeguarding the drugs, preventing pilferage, addiction and/or trafficking, and in this connection it is well to refer to the strong representations made by the League of Nations...regarding extra precautions necessary in war time to prevent a repetition of the unfortunate state of affairs arising through the last war.[9]

The proliferation of drug use during the First World War had left an indelible imprint on the drug control apparatus, both globally and nationally. Indeed, the over-riding fear of governments was that the great expansion in addiction that occurred during and after the first global conflict would be replicated in the second. The 'strong representations' made by the League were, in fact, principally responsible for the continued existence of the Drugs Branch following the outbreak of hostilities in September 1939. In its Annual Report for 1941, the Branch had observed that:

> On the outbreak of War and at the urgent request of the League of Nations it was decided that the work of the Drugs Branch should continue in view of the fact that the present control was instituted after the last War because during the War period addiction to, and traffic in, habit forming drugs had assumed such proportions as to cause serious alarm in most countries of the world. The importance of maintaining this control during the present War could scarcely be overemphasised.[10]

[9] TNA HO 45/21172, Thornton to Harris 18 April 41.
[10] TNA HO 45/24948, Drugs Branch Annual Report for 1941.

Despite this commitment, the wartime government cut back severely on the Branch's personnel.[11] The number of dangerous drugs inspectors was reduced by half, and at one point in early 1941, the entire Drugs Branch consisted solely of Frank Thornton and a couple of typists. While its perennial struggle with script doctors continued, much of the Branch's wartime work was directly influenced by the circumstances of the conflict, in particular as a consequence of the prominent role played by the Home Front following Dunkirk. The Branch was responsible for ensuring sufficient drug supplies were available for all the requirements of the Home Front. It reported that it had, 'in consultation with the Ministry of Health...arranged the purchase, storage and supervision of a large quantity of Raw Opium for Government Reserve Stock', to be deployed in the manufacture of morphine.[12] In addition, the Drugs Branch negotiated with manufacturers for the setting up of 'shadow factories' for morphine production, thereby ensuring the nation's wartime supply. Most directly, the Branch was forced to relocate its offices from the capital to the relative tranquillity of Bournemouth on the south coast of England after the Home Office suffered a bomb damage in which some of Thornton's own paperwork had been buried.[13]

Structural and Legislative Reorganisation of the Nation's Health

Like much of Britain's social and economic infrastructure, health services were reorganised when the Second World War broke out.[14] The Civil Defence Act of 1939 permitted the introduction of the emergency medical services, giving the state power to direct both municipal and voluntary

[11] During the 1930s, its optimum staffing level consisted of four inspectors, a staff officer and several clerical and administrative staff. In the advent of war, Chief Inspector William Coles was himself transferred to the Ministry of Labour and National Service, although he continued to take an interest in drugs affairs and gave advice when necessary. Boothroyd, another inspector, was called up for national service, leaving Frank Thornton and John Sloane, and the latter was, for reasons which remain unclear, 'summarily dismissed' in January 1941. The Branch was able to recruit a very able new inspector in the form of Len Dyke, who had, in the late 1930s, been the leading expert drugs officer at Scotland Yard, though he was unable to take up the Drugs Branch post until April 1941. This left Thornton as the sole member of Britain's Home Office Drugs Branch for a period of three months.

[12] HO 45/24948, Home Office Drugs Branch, Annual Report 1941.

[13] MH 76/83, Thornton to Neville, 26 April 1941.

[14] R. M. Titmuss, *Problems of Social Policy* (Basingstoke: Palgrave Macmillan, 2002).

hospitals and incorporating them into the Emergency Hospital Scheme.[15] In order to prevent hospitals becoming overwhelmed by casualties, particularly from air attack, a layered system was established. Casualties would be handled by three main levels of medical response: First Aid Posts, Mobile Units and hospitals. The First Aid Posts were intended to treat the 'walking wounded', those suffering from minor injuries and shock; each post had a doctor assigned. The Mobile Units generally consisted of trucks converted and equipped for emergency medicine, which could attend incidents as required. The hospitals were, meanwhile, reserved for the more serious cases.[16]

While ARP had had an institutional existence since 1924, it was after the 1935 announcement that Germany was rearming the Luftwaffe that a specific ARP department was launched as a section of the Home Office.[17] Its aims were threefold: to maintain the morale of the people in the face of air attack, to ensure that essential services remained functional and to reduce the damage to life and property caused by air raids.[18] The first priority of ARP, then, was to maintain morale; adequate access to morphine was viewed by many doctors as integral to achieving this objective. As the war approached, the Home Office oversaw First Aid Posts, while the Ministry of Health bore responsibility for ambulances, hospitals and mortuaries. The relationship between the Home Office and the Ministry of Health was already marked by fluctuating degrees of acrimony, with, as Berridge has shown, differences of direction and emphasis in respect to drug policy stretching back to the post-Great War period.[19] The Home Office had originally insisted First Aid Posts should be staffed by lay personnel, with no doctor present. The medical profession had disputed this fiercely; in the House of Commons, Sir Francis Fremantle, himself a doctor and chairman of the Parliamentary Medical Committee, argued in November 1938 that 'first-aid posts would be perfectly useless without a

[15] G. Rivett, *The Development of the London Hospital System, 1823–1982* (Oxford: Oxford University Press, 1986).

[16] 'Air Raid Casualty Services', *British Medical Journal* 2,4168 (1940) pp. 716–7. Later, these were supplemented by light units consisting of a car carrying a doctor and nurse.

[17] R. Mackay, *Half the Battle: Civilian Morale in Britain During the Second World War* (Manchester: Manchester University Press, 2002) p. 31.

[18] Ibid.

[19] Berridge, *Opium and the People*, pp. 258–278.

medical officer'.[20] Following the Munich crisis, the problems of coordination amongst the Ministry of Health, the Home Office, the local authorities and the medical profession were felt to be so serious that a joint deputation from the British Medical Association, the Royal College of Physicians and the Royal College of Surgeons was dispatched to lobby the Minister for the Coordination of Defence. This political and professional advocacy was effective, and responsibility for First Aid Posts was reassigned to the Ministry of Health, which took care to include supplies of morphine.[21] This change in approach was largely because, aside from any general differences in orientation between the two departments, the medical community possessed a much greater sensitivity toward the psychological effects of attack from the air, having spent several years engaged in debates surrounding civilian hysteria and neurosis, which, it was anticipated, would accompany air raids.[22]

In comparison with the First World War, the Second saw remarkably little legislative and regulatory change with regard to drugs. The sole exception was the legislation governing their use by hospitals.[23] The Hospital General Exemption Order of 1924 permitted hospitals to possess dangerous drugs for use on individual patients in accordance with the prescription of a medical practitioner. This arrangement was changed by an amendment order in August 1939, permitting hospitals to possess and supply drugs 'otherwise than for the treatment of individual patients in the hospital', that is, at First Aid Posts and so on.[24] The passing of the amendment provided an early indication that the problematic relationship obtaining between the Home Office and the Ministry of Health in the 1920s had endured. In the build-up to war, the Ministry had arranged to use the London County Council as its buying agent for the Emergency Hospital Scheme in the London area, and the Council was poised to pur-

[20] Hansard, 30.11.1938 p. 511 Fremantle also reminded the House that 'that in an air raid you might not only have numbers of the civil population wounded, but you might have a large number of medical cases among the civil population—cases of nervous breakdown, hysteria, mania, and mental cases—with which it would be very difficult to deal'.

[21] TNA HO 45/21172, Thornton to Harris 18 April 1941.

[22] Mackay, *Half the Battle*, pp. 31–38.

[23] HO 45/25377, 'Administration of morphine to air raid casualties'; memorandum by Thornton, 25 April 1951. In this note, Thornton confirms (in the course of a discussion of postwar requests to produce legislation permitting the use of morphine by civil defence staff) the fact that no other drugs legislation was introduced during the Second World War.

[24] TNA HO 45/19807, Dangerous Drugs (Hospital General Exemption) (Amendment) Order (1939).

chase some 83 kilogrammes of morphine sulphate for the scheme when a major legal hurdle became apparent.[25] According to Major Coles, writing shortly before the outbreak of war: 'The Ministry of Health made all their arrangements and only consulted me at the last moment when the London County Council expressed some doubt as to whether they were authorised under the Dangerous Drugs legislation to carry out the proposed transaction.'[26]

The other significant document was produced by the Ministry of Health in the form of an emergency medical circular. This was probably the most important of numerous circulars issued by the Ministry with respect to the handling of dangerous drugs in wartime but did not amend either the drug laws or the detailed regulations that enabled them to function. Rather, as discussed below, it was intended to cover certain practical problems arising in the course of the war.

Interdepartmental Wrangling over Morphine at First Aid Posts

In the months prior to the outbreak of hostilities, the Ministry of Health and the Home Office engaged in a fractious debate regarding the provision of dangerous drugs at First Aid Posts. The Ministry suggested that lay individuals such as ARP workers should be able to administer morphine, and approached the Home Office regarding the possibility of amending the legislation to allow this.[27] Thornton noted that 'in the past the medical profession had expressed very strong views against the administration of dangerous drugs by laymen' but that the Ministry's medical experts 'have now decided that in wartime such use by laymen will be essential'.[28] Typical of the practitioners' views was a letter from a Dr Hamill of London W1, which appeared in both *The Lancet* and the *British Medical Journal* and argued that, owing to the shortage of skilled staff at First Aid Posts and Mobile Units, 'it is essential that all voluntary assistants should be trained to administer morphine by hypodermic injection'.[29]

[25] TNA HO 45/19807, Drugs to be ordered by LCC under Emergency Hospital Scheme, n.d.

[26] TNA HO 45/19807, Cover notes by Major Coles.

[27] TNA HO 45/21172, Thornton to Coles, 19 April 1939.

[28] TNA HO 45/21172, Drugs Branch to Logan, Ministry of Health, 25 April 1939.

[29] P. Hamill, 'Morphine Injection at First Aid Posts' Lancet 233,6038 (1939) pp. 1139–1192. See also *British Medical Journal* 1,4089 (1939) p. 1054.

According to the Ministry of Health, there were around 3200 First Aid Posts scattered across the country.[30] In order to obtain a picture of the conditions prevailing with respect to the handling of drugs at these posts, the Home Office carried out inspections in a number of London boroughs in late 1939. A total of 12 posts were inspected in 10 boroughs, the resulting report stating that: 'The position is the same in all with the partial exception of Mitcham, namely that Dangerous Drugs are readily available to sundry persons at the First Aid Posts.'[31] The report continued that the position was 'extremely serious since the theft or loss of drugs at any particular post is all that is required to create a first class scandal. Considerable laxity seems to have been shown by all Medical Officers of Health in not realising the true position with regard to the drugs covered by the Dangerous Drugs Regulations'.[32] Medical Officers of Health were targeted for these criticisms because they had been assigned overall responsibility for the drugs they delivered to medics at local First Aid Posts. The Home Office called for a circular to be produced by the Ministry and sent out to all Medical Officers of Health to remind them of their duties under the regulations, and the two departments collaborated on its drafting.[33] As the authority responsible for regulating dangerous drugs, the Home Office held the upper hand in the negotiations, and adopted a position in which the central concern was to restrict the access to drugs of addicts and citizens, the latter whom it viewed as potential addicts. It was preoccupied with the bureaucratic question of recording all drugs that went into this system; the dominant issue for those in the field, on the other hand, consisted in ensuring that morphine was available to the wounded—even if a doctor could not be present.

The resulting circular was entitled 'Storage of Dangerous Drugs at First Aid Posts', and it was sent out to County Medical Officers and Medical Officers of Health and to local authorities. It explained that the Home Office had approached the Minister of Health regarding 'the importance of ensuring the safe custody of dangerous drugs issued as part of the medical equipment of First Aid Posts, and for securing that proper supervision is exercised in their administration'.[34] The circular concluded by acknowl-

[30] Ibid.

[31] TNA HO 45/21172, Memo 'First Aid Posts' 09 November 1939.

[32] Ibid.

[33] Ibid.

[34] TNA HO 45/21172, Ministry of Health circular 'Storage of Dangerous Drugs at First Aid Posts' 05 January 1940.

edging, though in terms that were less than explicit, the key point around which the problem coalesced: that there might be occasions on which the post's doctor—or any doctor—was unable to personally attend an emergency. It recommended that the Medical Officer of Health or County Medical Officer retain a duplicate key to the post's dangerous drugs cabinet.[35] However, no stipulation was made as to who was to be allowed access to this duplicate key and, by implication, who would control and utilise the supplies of morphine. When this point was raised, the Home Office had 'semi-officially' suggested that a spare key be kept at the premises in a glass case that could be broken under emergency conditions.[36] However, it still failed to identify the steps to be taken if authorised medical personnel were unavailable—and who was to take them. The assumption appeared to be that some other doctor would be available if the one assigned to the post was elsewhere; but such an assumption was unrealistic. The circular missed its objective, insofar as it failed to acknowledge the conditions likely to prevail in actual air raid conditions, when it was probable that none of the medics mentioned by the circular, or the 'semi-official' equivocations that followed it, would be present at the post; many were responsible for more than one facility, and senior figures often covered large geographical areas. The situation was particularly acute in remote rural regions.

Mackenzie of the Department of Health for Scotland contended that the demands of medical treatment and the maintenance of morale possessed greater urgency and importance than strict obedience to the dangerous drugs regulations. Fraser of the Ministry of Health made a similar point, reminding Thornton by letter in March 1941 that 'the doctor is not always the first on the scene'.[37] Thornton told the Ministry that, according to the Home Office interpretation of the dangerous drugs regulations, 'The law does not allow morphia to be given out...in advance. There must be an actual and not merely a hypothetical patient to be treated.'[38] Posited in this way, it was difficult to see how it would ever be possible for wounded people to be treated within the law in situations where no doctor was either present or accessible. It is this point on which the circular was intended to provide definitive advice, but which it effectively sidestepped.

[35] Ibid.

[36] TNA HO 45/21172, Thornton to Mackenzie 30 January 1940.

[37] TNA HO 45/21172, Fraser to Thornton, 24 March 1941.

[38] TNA MH 76/83, Bearn to Harris, 21 July 1941.

There were many complaints made by doctors working on the Home Front regarding the proliferation of circulars emanating from the Ministry of Health. '(R)running into several hundred', these circulars 'flooded' the profession and as a result 'were not treated with the attention which they should be'.[39] Partly for this reason and partly because the 'Storage of Dangerous Drugs' circular had evaded the central issue, its message failed to have much impact on the ground. Numerous cases of regulatory transgressions or potential transgressions continued to come to Home Office attention.

Morphia and National Morale

Underpinning the unease felt by the medical profession was a pervasive belief amongst doctors that the emergency conditions flowing from air raids would overwhelm the medical profession's ability to attend casualties and provide adequate levels of pain relief. It was feared that the proliferation of suffering and untended wounds would exacerbate the already devastating effect that aerial bombing was anticipated to have on civilian morale, producing outbreaks of feminised 'hysteria'.

This discourse is illustrated by the example of Dr Lankester, which 'Len' Dyke (then a Metropolitan Police officer) uncovered during a chemists' shop inspection in April 1940, just a few months after the circular had been issued. This doctor had prescribed large supplies of Omnopon and morphine 'for use in ARP work' at the post located in the Ministry of Agriculture and Fisheries in Whitehall.[40] It is significant that even here, in the heart of the government district, confusion prevailed concerning the regulation of morphine. Dyke informed the pharmacy manager that under the terms of the Acts, the ARP team was not unauthorised to possess these drugs.[41] Dr Lankester could not legally prescribe them for general use in ARP duties; he could prescribe only for an actual patient.

Dr Lankester explained that in the event of air attack, 'the first thing people would require would be either a tablet or an injection of morphia, etc. and to this end he had "stocked" the post in question and had left the drugs in charge of Patmore and other members of the ARP'.[42] He then

[39] TNA HO 45/21172, Thornton to Symon 21 December 1939.
[40] Omnopon was a medicine containing morphine and several other opiates.
[41] TNA HO 45/21172, CID Memo 01 May 1940.
[42] Ibid.

'reluctantly' confessed that the same procedure had been carried out at a number of other posts to which he was assigned. He further admitted that he kept no register of these, and, observed Dyke with some understatement, 'when closely questioned on the matter, was obviously not too well informed as to his position or the requirements of the regulations'.[43] Dyke commented: 'I said to Dr Lankester that his procedure according to law was entirely wrong and that dangerous drugs should not be permitted to be used in the manner described.'[44] The doctor's justification of his actions invoked images of wounded civilians and hysterical girls and the threat to morale that they posed. According to Dyke's notes:

> Dr Lankester declared that he appreciated the position really, but added the Authorities seemed to have overlooked the fact that if serious air raids did occur then hundreds of people and young girls in particular would be confined in basements... and to prevent "mass hysteria" he advocated the use of morphia and Omnopon injections or oral tablets and was quite prepared for these injections etc. to be in the care of "experienced" people who were admittedly not medical men.[45]

This practitioner argued that the Home Office officials should give some further consideration to his views, because 'in spite of the interview he was still of the opinion that, before thinking of rules and regulations the welfare of the people must come first'.[46]

Dyke observed that, 'Doctor Lankester, although perfectly frank in his replies, is obviously not too well acquainted with his position as a practitioner, in relation to "Dangerous Drugs". In addition, he has decided views of his own regarding the administration of drugs during air raids and his chief concern in this direction is to prevent "mass hysteria".'[47] Thornton added that, 'The man in charge of a first aid post might, in the excitement, be tempted to administer morphine to every girl who started to cry.'[48]

The assumption of a feminine subject here is significant; while the fear of panic under air attack was associated with civilians generally, it applied

[43] Ibid.
[44] Ibid.
[45] Ibid.
[46] Ibid.
[47] Ibid.
[48] Ibid.

to women in a specific, medically authorised way.[49] Thornton also noted that the doctor had declared himself prepared to administer opiates for cases of hysteria even where no physical injury was present. In fact, such willingness was not confined to Dr Lankester, but common in much of the medical profession, including amongst senior figures. The Home Office believed that 'the current sentiment of doctors is very much in favour of permitting unauthorised persons to be in charge of Dangerous Drugs at First Aid Posts'.[50] It concluded that 'this storage of drugs throughout the country in First Aid Posts has already led to a slackening on the part of doctors in their views regarding the administration of such drugs'.[51]

Illicit Access to Stockpiles of Opiates

What the Home Office saw as a 'slackening' of medical attitudes, considerable numbers of medical men viewed as a pragmatic and flexible response to an emergency. Whatever the perspective, did the enhanced presence of morphine in British society and the contextual problems involved in applying strict controls to it lead to increased nonmedical use? The Drugs Branch certainly thought so. Its correspondence with doctors and other government departments bristles with references to the attempts of opiate addicts to insinuate themselves into the mechanisms of civil defence in order to access the abundant stores of morphine now lodged there. A couple of examples should suffice to demonstrate the tone of the department's concern, the first being drawn from Thornton's correspondence with Mackenzie:

> (W)e have on record cases in which convicted criminals and also known drug addicts were engaged on A.R.P. work, so...you will appreciate that risks of loss or pilferage are far greater than they are in a chemist's shop or a doctor's house...you will see that we are not attempting to deal with 'out-and-out' burglary or theft but only with pilferage and drug possession brought about by the temptation presented to unqualified persons by easy access.[52]

[49] G. Swanson, *Drunk with the Glitter: Space, consumption and sexual instability in modern urban culture* (Abingdon & New York: Routledge, 2007) pp. 15–26.

[50] TNA HO 45/21172. Memo re. Dr Charles White, 05 March 1940.

[51] Ibid.

[52] TNA HO 45/21172, Thornton to Mackenzie 08 January 1940.

The internal discussions of the Drugs Branch also refer to cases of addict infiltration and disappearing drugs, with Thornton informing his Home Office superior, Sydney Harris, that, '...we have learned of several cases of loss and pilferage, and in a few cases some of our well-known London addicts have taken up A.R.P. or First Aid work!'.[53] One of these 'well-known London addicts' was Napper Dean Paul, who obtained a position with Kensington ARP thanks to his acquaintance with its head, Lord Cholmondeley.[54] Individuals like Paul probably found it a relatively simple matter to blend in with the general body of civil defence workers. Former actress and air raid warden Barbara Nixon commented on the social makeup of these services, observing that as those 'chancy means of livelihood closed down at the outbreak of war, there was a large percentage of bookie's touts, and even more parasitic professions, in the CD services, together with a mixed collection of workers in light industry, "intellectuals", opera singers, street traders, dog fanciers...chorus girls' and so on.[55,56] Such a milieu represented something close to the natural habitat of those West End lifers and bohemians from which the period's drug subculture was made up.

Addicts amongst nurses and doctors represented a particular problem for the wartime regulation of morphine due to their professional knowledge and qualifications and the privileged access to drugs these gave them. In September 1943, the *Daily Mirror* reported an example of the methods used to exploit the context of national emergency in order to support an opiate dependence.[57] Maud Brown, a nurse who prior to the German invasion of the Channel Islands had lived in Jersey and was, according to the police, a 'confirmed drug addict', had been 'sacked from a number of institutions' at which she worked on the British mainland. The dismissals allegedly occurred as a result of her drug use. Her latest escapade, which resulted in a court appearance, involved an initially successful endeavour to relieve the 'mental colony' at which she was employed of its stocks of morphine and heroin. Brown's method had been to initiate a false air raid alert, causing the institution to switch off its lighting; raiding the danger-

[53] TNA HO 45/21172, Thornton to Harris 18 April 1941.

[54] TNA MEPO 3/2579, CID Memo, 15 October 1941.

[55] B. Nixon, *Raiders Overhead: A Diary of the London Blitz* (London: Scolar Press, 1980) p. 82.

[56] An account of bohemian life in frontline London may be found in R. Hewison, *Under Siege: Literary Life in London 1939–1945* (Newton Abbott: Readers Union, 1978).

[57] *Daily Mirror*, 7 September 1943, p. 1.

ous drugs cabinet under the cover of darkness, she had made off with its heroin supplies. It was precisely the type of addict subterfuge that the Home Office dreaded.[58]

Dr Aymer Douglas Maxwell had meanwhile been struck off the medical register by the GMC in 1936 following a long series of regulatory transgressions. A confirmed morphine addict, his authority to possess dangerous drugs was withdrawn by the Home Secretary in 1935 after a host of offences and prescribing irregularities, but he continued to obtain supplies from London pharmacies despite his lack of authorisation.[59] Maxwell came to Home Office attention once again in 1942 in the context of discussions over the regulation of morphine at Royal Ordnance Factories. As these were vital spaces for the national defence, they could reasonably be expected to come under attack in the event of enemy invasion and were permitted both an on-site armoury and a First Aid Post stocked with adequate supplies of painkilling drugs. In an exchange regarding the adequacy of safeguards at these institutions, Coles made an interesting aside to Thornton: 'Did you know that Munro took on A.D. Maxwell as a medical officer in a Royal Ordnance Factory but he had to get rid of him after a period because of the old trouble.'[60] The 'old trouble' was, of course, morphine addiction, and Maxwell had taken up the position in order to enable him to access the factory's morphine supplies. Throughout the war, the Drugs Branch fought an ongoing battle with those who sought to gain illicit access to the nation's enhanced supply of drugs.

The cases recorded by the Home Office and those few that appeared in newspaper reports do not indicate that drug use was proliferating as it had in the previous world war. They mostly involved, as the Drugs Branch acknowledged, 'well-known addicts', and no cases of large-scale trafficking involving stocks assembled against war contingencies have come to

[58] While Maud Brown is a name that has not been encountered previously in this research, it is possible that there may have been a linkage with Brenda Dean Paul, who had lived in Jersey for some months in late 1938. In such a restricted geographical and social setting, a shared interest in opiates may well have drawn the two women together, particularly since Paul was a figure of such notoriety. However, the connection remains purely speculative at this stage.

[59] TNA HO 144/20168 gives full account of Maxwell's addict career. See also *British Medical Journal*, 2,3961, Supplement to the General Medical Council, 5 December 1936.

[60] HO 144/20168, The 'Munro' mentioned in connection with the employment of Dr Munro is Sir David Munro, Senior Medical Officer to the Ministry of Supply during the Second World War.

light, which was the Home Office's major concern. Against this backdrop, there seems scant justification for the Home Office's continual blocking of measures to alleviate the suffering of civilians. Its institutional perception of the situation was formed in the course of its two decades of law enforcement-centred drug control, summed up by Thornton in his comment that:

> Far too much trouble has been caused in the past by ready access to these drugs. The temptation to 'try everything once' is very strong in the average person, and in addition there are the risks of "trafficking" or "passing on" to willing purchasers when it becomes generally known that these drugs are available in the hands of unqualified persons.[61]

At the same time, it is arguable that there was some increase in nonmedical use during the years of the conflict, and the early development of a new phase of drug subculture. In Britain's years of postwar austerity and the mid-1950s postwar period of affluence associated with the rise of consumer society, new addict networks emerged, centred—initially at least—on a new wave of modernist jazz known as bebop. The music critic John Fordham, who was an intimate spectator of the growth of the bebop jazz scene in London, dates the beginnings of this new drug subculture to the war years and the bottle parties of the West End.[62] With large numbers of US servicemen for whom drug use was familiar, the proximity of sudden death, with

> the anxiety and exhilaration, and the long hours, came drugs.[63] The clubs were like sweetshops; variations of speed and heart stimulants intended for servicemen at the end of their tether, Benzedrine inhalers dismembered and dropped into teacups, marijuana. Availability and adventurousness were leading a new generation to experiment with narcotics seriously for the first time in Britain.[64]

[61] TNA HO 45/21172, Thornton to Harris 01 August 1941.

[62] According to painter Michael Wishart, who visited the nightclub scene as a teenager during the early war years, 'These clubs were about the only places where it was easy to buy marijuana, decades before it became the stock- in-trade of a generation.' See M. Wishart, *High Diver: An Autobiography* (London: Quartet, 1978) p. 24.

[63] This can be seen in the attitudes to the use of marijuana on display in the classic 1944 film by Michael Powell and Emeric Pressburger, *A Canterbury Tale*.

[64] J. Fordham, *Let's Join Hands and Contact the Living: Ronnie Scott and His Club* (London: Elm Tree Books, 1986) pp. 13–14. For the use of stimulants amongst the commercial sex workers of Soho in the 1940s, see also B. Tate, *West End Girls: The real lives, loves and friendship of 1940s Soho and its working girls* (London: Orion Books, 2010).

Although the present research has demonstrated that serious experimentation with narcotics had in fact begun much earlier, and despite the relative paucity of empirical evidence left by the period, I find Fordham's argument plausible. The war years were claimed by further authorities to have left a particular mark on the drug subculture. An unnamed member of the staff at Spelthorne St Mary's, for example, noted of the women clients who attended the convent's nursing home at this time that, in addition to acquiring drugs from both doctors and illicit sources, '(t)hese patients are usually of a dissipated and somewhat degraded type with no desire for a permanent cure. They come to have the drug tapered, and frequently leave before withdrawal is complete, and return to their habits needing a smaller amount to give the satisfaction they crave. This type of patient has greatly increased during the war'.[65] The extent to which the war impacted upon drug subcultural developments remains to be seen; the argument made in this section must remain tentative until such time as further research identifies a more substantial empirical evidence base. In broader historical terms, however, there is no doubt that postwar drug subcultures built upon trends that had been developing for several decades.

The Growth of Wartime Pragmatism at the Home Office

From the point of view of casualties, it was no doubt fortunate that an ethic of pragmatism prevailed in the delivery of services by medical teams who had learned their techniques in the course of their work. This was summed up by A. W. Neville, assistant secretary at the Ministry of Health, who conducted much of the Ministry's negotiations with the Home Office in regard to the question of morphine: 'Although the Circular does not, and could not, say that the drugs are to be administered by the nurse in an emergency, it gives abroad hint in that direction. What is supposed to happen under the Dangerous Drugs Acts and what actually happens in dire emergency are not necessarily the same thing....'[66] The Ministry of Health did contemplate taking the conflict with the Home Office further, but had learned that it could operate adequately on the 'nod and wink' principle referred to by Neville, making use of the 'broad hint' that, in the absence

[65] A Member of the Community of St Mary the Virgin, 'The Moral, Mental and Physical Background of Female Inebriates' *British Journal of Inebriety* 42,1 (1944) pp. 3–20.

[66] TNA MH 76/83, Note from Neville to Fraser 05 March 1941.

of a doctor, a nurse or somebody else would provide pain relief to those in need.[67] The Home Office would itself, in due course, come quietly to adopt this pragmatism.

The Ministry was moved to raise the issue again subsequent to one of the most potentially serious instances of the absence of pain relief for wounded civilians in January 1941, when the large public shelter at Bank underground station received a direct hit, severing contact between the shelter and the surface and killing in excess of 100 people.[68] In the event, a foreign medic happened by sheer good fortune to be present and was able to attend to the worst of the injuries by recourse to morphine supplies carried in his medical bag; however, this was clearly not a matter that could be left to chance.[69]

'Ministers are somewhat exercised in their minds as to what would happen as to the administration of morphia to civilians wounded in an emergency, if medical officers were not at hand when required', wrote Professor Fraser to Thornton within weeks of the events at Bank.[70] Edward Bearn, undersecretary at the Ministry of Health, pointed out to the Home Office that 'speaking generally the medical aid posts (in underground shelters) are each in charge of a doctor who visits...regularly once a night but then goes home and does not attend the shelter again that night unless on call'.[71] In the case of large public shelters, the Ministry argued, the Home Office suggestions failed to meet the problems posed by the bloody realities of the conflict. Bearn continued:

> The casualties which might occur...could be extremely serious and I am sure that you will agree that it would seem indefensible that human beings should be kept for hours in a state of intense suffering because of failure to find some way to meet special war time circumstances.[72]

In this setting, the Home Office response that a doctor could be sent out for or could relay his instructions was clearly inadequate. Bearn's detailed letter and his repeated invocation of the presence of the Minister—mixed no doubt with a generalised awareness across the state of

[67] TNA HO 45/21172, Bearn to Harris 21 July 1941.
[68] J. Gardiner, *Wartime: Britain 1939–1945* (London: Headline, 2004) p. 412.
[69] TNA HO 45/21172, Memorandum by Thornton, 19 August 1941.
[70] TNA HO 45/21172, Fraser to Thornton, 24 March 1941.
[71] TNA HO 45/21172, Bearn to Harris 21 July 1941.
[72] TNA MH 76/83, Bearn to Harris 21 July 1941.

the potential significance for national morale of what had taken place at Bank—produced the desired result, and it was decided 'to add a small quantity of morphine solution' to the equipment held at the large public air raid shelters.[73] Arrangements were made with London Underground to store supplies in a locked cupboard in the booking office during the day, and they would be held by a qualified nurse at night when the shelter was in use.

The Ministry of Health had pushed for first aid workers to carry morphine supplies, meeting with Home Office officials in May 1941. The early Home Office response was summarised by Thornton, who stated that 'we might as well dispense with the control of drugs forthwith, since quite an appreciable proportion of the public would be involved, and if they were to be allowed to be in more or less unsupervised possession of drugs, undesirable results would be bound to result'.[74]

In time, however, an increasingly pragmatic attitude from the Home Office allowed flexibility to be applied in other contexts where access to morphine was recognised to be essential. Debates surrounding regulation of dangerous drugs in the event of a German invasion grew throughout the remainder of 1941 and reached their peak in the ensuing year, indicating that the prospect of enemy landings by sea or parachute still occupied the attentions of Britain's civil servants long after Dunkirk and the 'Spitfire summer'.[75] The terms of the discussions remained essentially the same as those surrounding the provision of morphine to First Aid Posts, as did the lack of clarity amongst parts of the medical profession. There were cases where doctors took it on themselves to authorise nurses to possess and administer morphine, as in the case of Dr Hollins, attached to the East Sussex Home Guard.[76] The St Pancras Borough Council Medical Officer of Health, meanwhile, declared in September 1940 that it was now 'understood that the Medical Officer of Health should consider himself at liberty to modify somewhat the strict legal interpretation of the law in order to

[73] TNA MH 76/83, London Civil Defence Region Memo, 08 August 1941.

[74] TNA HO 45/21172, Thornton memo 20 May 1941.

[75] M. Donnelly, *Britain in the Second World War* (London: Routledge, 1999).

[76] TNA MH 76/83, Dr Clegg to Ministry of Health 19.06.1941. Dr Hollins was medical officer of the 22nd Battalion, Home Guard. He visited all the First Aid Posts in his area to advise them to buy morphine, at their own expense; he also wrote to District Nurses instructing them to administer morphine to casualties on their own initiative.

meet these very special circumstances'.[77] It was his intention henceforth to distribute morphine to stretcher parties attending bombed buildings—a suggestion that drew a hostile response from the Ministry, under Home Office guidance.[78] In view of the situation on the ground, therefore, the 'by the book' attitude of the Home Office was never likely to prevail, and the Ministry was able to issue a circular in December 1941 which permitted the administration of morphine by District Nurses.[79] It was designed to provide guidance and authority in villages or other rural districts which had been cut off under invasion conditions, where casualties required treatment yet no authorised medical practitioner could reach the site. At the sounding of 'Action Stations' or where invasion was imminent or taking place, stocks of morphine held by County Medical Officers of Health and reserved for the purpose were to be supplied to District Nurses. The measure was surrounded by various requirements, notably that the nurse could only administer only a 1.0 cc dose, which was judged to be too little to occasion an overdose. It was also felt necessary to stipulate that the Medical Officer may only provide the drugs to a District Nurse whom 'he knows to be trustworthy for the purpose'.[80]

In March 1942, the number of people authorised (though neither by the dangerous drugs laws nor the regulations made thereunder) to possess and administer morphine increased once again when it was extended to cover 'designated persons'. As before, these individuals were to be selected by Medical Officers of Health, though on what basis is not made explicit, except in vague terms. Fraser had scoffed at the notion that they would comprise 'the Vicar's wife' or the 'leading resident', the great and the good of county society.[81] Instead, it was urged that stocks should go to local police constables, Ministers of Religion, Home Guard Officers and equivalent representatives of authority.[82]

By the second year of conflict, pragmatism had begun to encroach on the bureaucratic citadel that was the Home Office and, by 1942, was explicit in its documentation. As Thornton put it in relation to the prospect of invasion: 'In such an event I feel that Regulations, Bye-laws,

[77] TNA MH 76/83, Maitland Radford to Air Raid Precautions Emergency Committee, 12 September 1940.

[78] TNA MH 76/83, Ministry of Health to St Pancras Town Hall, October 1940.

[79] TNA MH 76/83, Morphine for District Nurses, 26 December 1941.

[80] Ibid.

[81] TNA HO 45/21172, 'Distribution and use of morphine in invasion' 10 February 1942.

[82] TNA MH 76/83, Anderson to Neville, 18 February 1942.

Control, etc.etc. will, more or less, have to go by the board, and we should, in the interests of humanity, be forced to agree to almost any direct or indirect breach of the Dangerous Drugs legislation.'[83] This may appear an extraordinary admission from a lifelong bureaucrat committed to the strict control of drugs, and doubtless it is; however, it should be viewed as a reflection of the seriousness of the situation that Britain was perceived to be facing in early 1942. Thornton had informed Harris of his belief that 'when invasion occurs…actual breaches of the Dangerous Drugs legislation will have to be overlooked entirely'.[84] In the same letter, he alluded to leaving the post-invasion details of morphine administration 'to the common sense of the persons concerned'.[85] Such a transformation in attitude appears at first sight to be an impressive *volte-face*, but in fact the pragmatism of the Drugs Branch had been building up during the course of the war. Its early intransigence was replaced incrementally by a more practical outlook in which the threat of some minor and probably temporary diffusion of addiction was placed alongside the global catastrophe facing the British state. In keeping with the tradition of the British System, the entire trajectory of the Home Office response to the unpredictability of the medical situation on the Home Front was made up of various forms of 'turning a blind eye' toward what it knew would be breaches of the regulations, accompanied by a 'semi-official' discourse of guidance in the form of hints and ambiguities.[86] In this way, the British System had, once again, demonstrated its 'Britishness'. It kept calm and carried on. By the early summer of 1943, when the fortunes of war had turned decisively against the Axis powers and the threat of invasion of the British Isles receded, the Ministry of Health initiated moves to reduce the quantities of morphine that had been distributed around the civil defence system. Supplies at First Aid Posts and so on remained initially unaffected; the retraction of drugs only applied in the case of those issued to remote villages where no doctor resided. Even here, owing to the dissatisfaction of local powers, supplies were to be collected and stored by County Medical Officers of Health, a tactic that permitted them to be re-distributed

[83] TNA HO 45/21172, Thornton to Harris, undated (851,312/55). Emphasis added.

[84] TNA HO 45/21172, Thornton to Harris 17 February 1942.

[85] Ibid.

[86] For example, Thornton's assurance that: '…the administration by of morphine by the nurse in the absence of the doctor and without his instructions would be irregular…in such circumstances…the Home Office would certainly raise no objection whatever to the administration by the nurse'. TNA HO 45/21172, Memo by Thornton, 19 August 1941.

should circumstances change again. A circular was finally produced in July 1943 announcing the collection of drug supplies, though exceptions were granted if there was no doctor in the vicinity who possessed stocks of morphine for use in emergencies, such as air raids.[87]

Addicts and the People's War

While pragmatism now reigned in some elements of UK drug policy, in others the response of the authorities grew more repressive. The country's therapeutic addicts continued to receive their prescribed doses without interruption and, provided they remained within the medicalised roles assigned to them by the 'British System', went largely unmolested by Home Office and the police. These addicts, by and large, remained 'invisible' during the conflict. The figure of the subcultural drug addict, by contrast, did not sit easily within the narrative of the People's War, with its theme of a national unity forged in the fires of the Home Front.[88] For these addicts, it was feared, accessing and consuming drugs would overwhelm any competing loyalty to the nation. It was an attitude exemplified by Jean Cocteau, who had allegedly greeted the outbreak of hostilities in September 1939 by asking, 'How will I get my opium?'.[89]

The Second World War saw the fortunes of Brenda Dean Paul follow a decisive downward arc; the lifestyle of hired Daimlers, luxury hotels and nightclubs was replaced by residence in seedy boarding rooms, disputes with her father over funds he refused to provide to meet the costs of 'cures', and even a court case in which Jean Baird, Paul's closest friend and lover in the late 1930s, testified against her for the unauthorised use of Baird's Harrods account to purchase a bottle of whisky and a few cosmetics.[90] It is impossible to disentangle Paul's personal descent from the social and cultural context of the Home Front, and the kind of informal treason addicts were understood to be perpetrating.

Prevalent attitudes are reflected in some of the representations produced by the British state to orchestrate civilian morale, perhaps the best example being the Ministry of Information poster, 'Keep mum, she's not

[87] TNA MH 76/83, EH Circular 70/43, 16 August 1943.

[88] S. O. Rose, *Which People's War? National Identity and Citizenship in Wartime Britain 1939–45* (Oxford: Oxford University Press, 2003).

[89] F. Steegmuller, *Cocteau: A Biography* (London: Constable, 1986) p. 436.

[90] *Times* 3 July 1939, p. 11; *Daily Mirror* 8 July 1939, p. 4; *Daily Express* 8 July 1939, p. 7.

so dumb' that formed part of the 'careless talk costs lives' series. Here, a woman of the 'femme fatale' type associated with nightlife, clubs, promiscuous sexual pleasure and intoxication—an image strongly redolent of figures such as Brenda Dean Paul, Bella Gold and Freda Roberts—is portrayed as a German agent or sympathiser. In the nightlife setting, surrounded by British officers who are drinking, smoking and chatting, she remains detached and watchful as she gathers (and, we are to assume, later passes on) information vital for Britain's national security.[91] Her gaze—knowing, conspiratorial—meets that of the viewer.

The social and cultural marginalisation of addicts was exemplified in the harsh sentences handed out to Paul during the war years, from a one-year prison sentence in April 1940 for various petty offences to a six months' sentence in November 1943 for heroin possession.[92] The social pressures Paul felt during this time persuaded her to change her name to Brenda Isolla Hampton in an attempt to escape the stigma with which she had become associated.[93]

The immediate postwar years of austerity saw limited evidence to support Home Office anxieties of cities awash with wartime drug supplies. Various cases of morphine supplies finding their way into illicit hands were reported, with instances of surplus war stocks including morphine supplies being sold to members of the public, in addition to thefts, probably quite widespread but involving small quantities, of the drug from several RAF bases.[94,95] Those larger-scale cases of opiates drawn from military stocks for trafficking purposes usually involved the US military, possibly because the quantities of drugs they held were, like everything else, more sizeable than their British equivalents; in 1952, 88 boxes of syrettes obtained from the US Army medical department were found following an arrest in East London, while 200 morphine doses were located in the possession of a

[91] Addicts seem to have been linked by reputation with the entire class of wartime undesirables—spivs, deserters, the wide classes, those who lived in 'funkholes' or hotels used as unofficial sanctuaries for individuals who were not inclined to national service and so on.

[92] TNA MEPO 3/2579, Return of Convictions recorded against Brenda Dean Paul, 17 November 1952.

[93] TNA MEPO 3/2579, CID Memo 12 May 1944.

[94] TNA HO 45/21934, Memorandum, A. L. Dyke 12 December 1947. This case was one in which military surplus lifeboats had been sold off to the public. Later it was discovered that the first aid kits these vessels carried were complete and included a quantity of morphine intended for maritime emergency.

[95] TNA HO 45/23161, Memo, Gloucestershire Constabulary 6 July 1948.

22-year-old labourer who claimed to be selling them on behalf of a corporal in the Canadian Army Medical Corps.[96] There is little doubt that further cases of such leakage of drugs into the nonmedical sphere went unrecognised by the authorities. However, the major source of drugs for the growing postwar opiate subculture continued to derive not from diverted civil defence sources but from the prescribing pads of script doctors and, to a lesser but gradually increasing extent, from thefts and forgeries that diverted them from the licit market and into the clubs and bars of the West End.

While it continued to pursue the same vicious addicts who had exercised it in the pre-war years, the Home Office was driven toward a more pragmatic approach by the Second World War. This was particularly the case with regard to medical professionals, who were—eventually—permitted to provide supplies to various lay people in order to alleviate pain and panic and to maintain civilian morale in the face of enemy air attack.

[96] TNA MEPO 3/2954, Annual Report of HMG to the League of Nations for 1952.

CHAPTER 8

Postwar Britain: Subcultural Transitions and Transmissions

Introduction

Following the double-stranded response of the Home Office to the years of conflict, which involved the continued campaign against the vicious addicts and the more relaxed outlook toward supplies for medical purposes, this chapter explores what has been called the 'postwar boom' in opiate addiction.[1] An expansion in the numbers using opiates—especially heroin—took place in the 1950s and 1960s, and has been seen as underpinning the demise of the classic British System of prescribing heroin to patients by general practitioners. The second Interdepartmental Committee, chaired by Lord Russell Brain and publishing its report in 1965, viewed the growth in addiction as the result of overprescribing by 'not more than six doctors', and led to a clinic-based system with only those doctors on the staff of the treatment centres permitted to supply heroin and cocaine to addicts.[2] Much of the academic research carried out on the period, usually by sociologists, has argued that the expansion in addict numbers, and more especially changes in the *type* of addicts, had brought about the policy changes that ended the Rolleston model.

[1] M. Kohn, *Narcomania: On Heroin* (London: Faber and Faber, 1987).

[2] Ministry of Health: Scottish Home and Health Department, *The Second Report of the Interdepartmental Committee on Drug Addiction* (London: HMSO, 1965) para.12. There were two governmental reports published within five years of each other in this period, both chaired by Russell Brain. The first appeared in 1961 and was tasked with reviewing the 1926 Rolleston Report. See Interdepartmental Committee on Drug Addiction *Report* (London: HMSO, 1961).

C. Hallam, *White Drug Cultures and Regulation in London, 1916–1960*, https://doi.org/10.1007/978-3-319-94770-9_8

However, these studies, while partly accurate, make various assumptions which access to recently opened archival resources has rendered problematic. The debates are examined below, and a modified argument proposed in which the transformations that characterised the postwar years are reassessed. As a result, I argue that the shifts in patterns of heroin use were not a matter of an opiate subculture appearing in place of the pre-war medicalised addicts, or of overprescribing script doctors taking over from normative practitioners. Rather, one wave of the UK's opiate subculture morphed into another, larger grouping, a group linked with the youth culture that came with the more developed consumer society of the 1950s. Elements within this youth subculture were attracted to the attitudes and practices of bohemianism and to a new wave of modernist jazz for which the figure of the outsider was personified in the heroin addict. In addition, the build-up of an established body of script doctors over previous decades provided the drug availability necessary for the proliferation of addiction, driving the market until the latter part of the 1960s when new illicit trafficking networks began to supply the UK market. Finally, it is notable that the development of this subculture was further supported by changes taking place from the 1940s onwards, when already there was a small but increasing criminal involvement in attempts to satisfy the domestic market for opiates and cocaine. This cluster of trends, events and identities enabled the growth of a new form of opiate subculture and will be examined below.

The Illicit Supply of Heroin in the 1940s

After the Second World War, the subcultural changes reported during the conflict continued, and a growth in illicit drug supplies was visible.[3] Of course, criminals had long sought to draw on the financial potential of illicit supply, but they had done so on an international scale, smuggling opiates to the USA through a network of European contacts. In Britain, a stream of relatively large-scale thefts and forgeries in the late 1940s and 1950s represented a new focus on the domestic market, and indicates a perception in the criminal underworld of the West End that the demand for illicit drugs, while still tiny compared to North American appetite, was now expanding.

Initially, there was an attempt to enlarge what was then the main domestic source of illicit supplies to nonmedical users—that deriving from

[3] These changes in attitude and behaviour are discussed in Chap. 7, pp. 226–227.

forged prescriptions. The first attempt to set up a systematic method for producing forged scripts took place in 1947, emerging from the criminal element of the West End life. The prime mover behind this attempt was Wilfred Cooper, who ran a Soho estate agency under the alias Tony Ross.[4] Cooper used his estate agent business to arrange accommodation for the sex industry and the 'marriage of convenience' racket that operated between London and the continent.[5] He had close links with the Montmartre district of Paris and may have been involved in cross-channel heroin traffic. Cooper himself had a heroin habit, as did Robert Clement, his lieutenant, who had run a nightclub in Fouberts Place in 1938 after the arrest of Gerry O'Brien.[6]

Cooper introduced several French associates to doctors who were known to him, having first provided them with forged letters of authorisation from physicians and/or government departments confirming their status as addicts and claiming that they had been in receipt of heroin and cocaine in either Paris or Dublin. These associates were not, in fact, using drugs, though some had done so in the past. The practitioners involved were Dr Marks Ripka, who had been a script doctor since 1935, and Dr John Oni Akerele, a Nigerian physician who intermittently supplied small numbers of addicts. However, both the Home Office and the Met believed that on these particular occasions both doctors were innocent victims of forgery. The heroin and cocaine obtained were probably sold on by Cooper; the scale of the operation points to this, as it outstrips any previous attempts at this kind of prescription forgery, which was usually intended purely for personal use. The sophisticated documentation required to authorise these supplies of heroin and cocaine, in addition to the quantities involved—1176 1/6th grain diamorphine tablets plus 440 1/2 grain cocaine hydrochloride tablets—marked Cooper's project off from the routine prescription forgery, as does the protagonists' entrenched

[4] TNA CRIM 1/1908, 'Defendant: Cooper, Wilfred and others. Charge: Conspiracy to contravene the Provisions of Regulation 2(1) of the Dangerous Drugs Act 1937, and unlawfully procuring drugs. 16 March 1948.' This case is also mentioned, though no names are given, in G. Lyle, 'Dangerous Drug Traffic in London' *British Journal of Addiction* 50,1 (1953) pp. 47–55.

[5] On the operation of the 'marriage of convenience' racket, which enabled foreign prostitutes to enter Britain and conferred upon them a level of protection against deportation, see S. Slater, 'Pimps, Police and Filles de Joie: Foreign Prostitution in Interwar London' *The London Journal*, 32,1 (2007) pp. 53–74.

[6] *Times* 16 March 1938, p. 9.

involvement in the transnational criminal underworld. This was, perhaps, the beginning, albeit on a minor scale, of the engagement of professional villains in the commercial retail supply of dangerous drugs in London.

In the ensuing years, there were at least four major thefts of opiates and cocaine from pharmaceutical manufacturers and wholesalers. Two of these resulted in prosecutions, the first being organised by Frederick Barnes, a 'coloured man', who made contact with several West End addicts, all allegedly known to the Home Office, and sold them morphine and cocaine.[7] Barnes was known on the street as 'Prince Frederick of Pakistan' while he distributed supplies amongst the addicts of the West End. Visiting the home of Maureen Brazil, he showed her a case full of morphine and cocaine and told her that 'These will make your mouth water'.[8] The perpetrators were eventually caught and given prison sentences, with Barnes receiving the longest at five years. None of the offenders were addicts and engaged in the venture on purely commercial grounds.

Dancing Mark and Advent of the London Heroin Subculture

While it has been discussed on previous occasions, the case of 'Mark', prosecuted for trafficking in 1951, has acquired an iconic status in the historiography of British heroin addiction and supply, and requires some comment in the context of this chapter.[9] 'Mark' was an alias used by Kevin Patrick Saunders, a young working-class man who had been employed as a porter at All Saints' Hospital in Chatham. After leaving his post at the hospital, Saunders returned to purloin a large quantity of morphine, cocaine and heroin from its stocks of dangerous drugs. He subsequently sold retail amounts of these drugs to customers in the West End of London—according to the *Daily Express*, these consumers were 'coloured men and their too-young-to-know girls'—and in so doing, he became 'the

[7] TNA HO 319/1, Dyke to Burley, 22 February 1960. The 'well-known addicts' included Jean Baird, Maureen Mary Brazil and possibly Brenda Dean Paul.

[8] *Daily Mirror* 5 May 1949, p. 1. See also *Daily Mail* 12 July 1949, p. 7.

[9] H. B. Spear, 'The Growth of Heroin Addiction in the United Kingdom' *British Journal of Addiction* 64, (1969) pp. 245–255; G. Lyle, 'Dangerous Drug Traffic in London' *British Journal of Addiction* 50, 1 (1953) pp. 47–55; H. F. Judson, *Heroin Addiction in Britain: What Americans can learn from the English experience* (London and New York: Harcourt Brace, 1974). P. Bean, *The Social Control of Drugs* (London: Wiley Blackwell, 1968). Numerous other works draw upon these sources.

mystery man that dancehall denizens called Dancing Mark and Scotland Yard's Narcotics Squad hunted for three months'.[10] Operating out of the clubs and coffee bars that had mushroomed in Soho to cater to the emergent youth culture, 'Mark' has been widely viewed as the 'source of infection' for a new network of addicts, which the Home Office was able to trace thanks to his helpful practice of maintaining a notebook which contained his customers' initials.[11] At the Drugs Branch, Spear compiled an epidemiological listing of 63 addicts whose addiction he traced, directly or indirectly, to the activities of Dancing Mark.[12] This inventory was of major importance in the narcotic historiography of twentieth-century Britain and is often viewed as marking the turning point from the medical addict to the opiate subculture.

At Saunders' court appearance, his own counsel described his activities as having helped 'to feed the stream of pollution which seems to be running though London'.[13] Such a construction was typical of the way in which drug cases were inserted into a wider narrative of metropolitan and national danger and decay. Frank Mort has elaborated this process with respect to postwar sexual delinquencies, but it applies with equal force to drugs.[14] During the ambivalent decade of the 1950s, the UK was undergoing a movement from the early postwar years of austerity toward a period of affluence, with an expanding menu of consumer goods and services that made available new types of food, sexual practices and, of course, drugs.[15] Drugs and commercial sex represented an illicit consumerism that

[10] *Daily Express* 18 October 1951, p. 5. In fact, the vast majority of Saunders' customers were white.

[11] H. F. Judson, *Heroin Addiction in Britain: What Americans can learn from the English experience* (London and New York: Harcourt Brace, 1974) pp. 28–29.

[12] H. B. Spear, 'The Growth of Heroin Addiction in the United Kingdom' *British Journal of Addiction* 64, (1969) pp. 245–255.

[13] *Daily Express* 18 October 1951, p. 5.

[14] A characteristic shared with sexual news events, as pointed out by Frank Mort. See F. Mort, *Capital Affairs: London and the Making of the Permissive Society* (New Haven & London: Yale University Press, 2010) p. 137.

[15] For discussion of the 1950s, see N. Thomas, 'Will the real 1950s please stand up? Views of a Contradictory Decade' *Cultural and Social History*, 5,2 (2008) pp. 227–236; B. Conekin, F. Mort, & C. Waters (eds) *Moments of Modernity: Reconstructing Britain 1945–1964* (London & New York: Rivers Oram Press, 1999); D. Kynaston, Austerity *Britain 1945–51* (London: Bloomsbury, 2007); D. Sandbrook, *Never Had It So Good: A History of Britain from Suez to the Beatles* (London: Brown, Little, 2006); A. Horn, *Juke Box Britain: Americanisation and youth culture, 1945–1960* (Manchester: University Press, 2009).

subtended the exuberant marketplace of the surface economy. While the tabloid press had in the immediate postwar period represented the flow of drugs as a part of a black market controlled by the wartime 'spiv', it was now viewed as the shadow of the 'bright lights' of opportunity and consumption in a capital inhabited by a significant new youth culture.[16] Most implicated in governmental anxieties aroused by these changes were the 'modern music clubs' of the West End. *The Times* recalled that one young teenager, a plumbers' mate arrested for supplying Indian hemp, had acquired his drug habits in precisely these spaces, where white girls were preyed upon by black men seeking sexual satisfaction and willing to use hemp drugs to obtain it.[17] The great fear of the state—that these drugs would spread from marginal ethnicities and the bohemian subculture to reach the irresponsible elements amongst the indigenous youth population—was apparently becoming a reality.

Soon after the trial of 'Mark', Detective Sergeant George Lyle informed a meeting of the Society for the Study of Addiction how, in order to track down Dancing Mark, the Met launched a young female detective named Catherine Arnold onto the streets of Soho dressed in the 'appropriate uniform of the "bebop" dancers, blue jeans and short haircut, etc.' to infiltrate Mark's circle of customers in 'the low clubs and cafes'.[18,19] These were the same undercover techniques that officers had made use of in the 1920s against the cocaine trade in the streets around Leicester Square and Soho. In his statement to the police, Saunders explained that having stolen the drugs, he headed for London to sell them. 'I approached a coloured man in the Charring Cross Road', he explained; the 'coloured man' had introduced him to other buyers. In Spear's epidemiological listing, only two subjects were addicts already known to the Drugs Branch: Barry Ellis and Angela Wyndham-Wilson. The presence of the other customers was newly recorded, though a few had previous cocaine and/or cannabis offences. Several later informed Spear that there was little or no heroin available in the West End prior to Saunders' appearance. Moreover, Spear remarks, Saunders' arrival coincided with a shortage of the newly popular cannabis due to enforcement pressures exerted on the area by the

[16] *Daily Mirror* 26 March 1947, p. 2.

[17] *Times*, 15 July 1957, p. 11.

[18] G. Lyle, 'Dangerous Drug Traffic in London' *British Journal of Addiction* 50,1 (1953) pp. 47–55.

[19] Ibid.

Met. Spear believed that the lack of cannabis propelled users toward heroin; in terms of further factors underlying the advent of this new group, meanwhile, Spear offers none.[20]

The Role of Doctors in the Postwar Boom

The advent of new heroin users in the 1950s has usually been constructed as an abrupt change, a subcultural break with a past landscape made up of compliant therapeutic addiction. Judith Blackwell claims that the 'handful of nontherapeutic opiate dependents living in Britain before 1950 could not have been said to constitute any sort of drug-using subculture'.[21] The new English heroin subculture of the 1950s and 1960s, she contends, was in fact a transatlantic phenomenon that arrived in postwar Britain along with the American discourse of the junkie outsider, associated with modernist or bebop jazz and the literature of the beat generation, and embedded in the street hustler lifestyle practised in the East Coast cities of the USA where heroin use had quickly re-established itself after the enforced abstinence of the war years. According to Blackwell, the 'sudden appearance of overprescribing physicians' in Britain was itself the result of this novel subculture which, in the absence of an illicit street market, sourced heroin and cocaine from doctors, among whom the addicts sought out the vulnerable and pressured them into providing prescriptions.[22] Blackwell's argument was deployed in contrast to the then widely accepted view that a small number of overprescribing doctors generated the new and expanded London drug scene in the late 1950s and early 1960s, forcing upon reluctant policy-makers the changes that ushered in the demise of classic British System. Her work is important and introduced into these debates a recognition of more complex cultural factors as well as an important international dimension.

However, as illustrated in previous chapters, this version of events does not always map comfortably onto the available evidence. The early post-Rolleston years were neither bereft of subcultural opiate-using groups nor marked by the absence of script doctors. Indeed, it was largely the

[20] H. B. Spear, 'The Growth of Heroin Addiction in the United Kingdom' *British Journal of Addiction* 64, (1969) pp. 245–255.

[21] J. Blackwell, 'The Saboteurs of Britain's Opiate Policy: Overprescribing Physicians or American-Style "Junkies"?' *The International Journal of the Addictions,* 23, (1988) pp. 517–526.

[22] Ibid. p. 524.

expansive and problematic prescribing of Dr Connor that drove the setting up of the Rolleston Committee. What was distinctive about the new wave of addiction in the 1950s was not its contrast with earlier decades of compliant medical addicts but rather that certain aspects of its social, cultural and demographic makeup differed from the pre-existing opiate subculture, mainly in terms of its age and its class makeup, though this latter would only fully take hold in the early 1960s. The changes were linked to developments in a much broader social field than that related specifically to drugs: the advent of new types of youth culture, the greater normative flexibility of postwar consumer Britain, the dissemination of bohemian discourses and lifestyles which took hold in certain strands of the youth culture and the build-up of a sufficient base of script doctors to provide expanded supplies of opiates to the market.

Although some level of underworld involvement in the illicit retail supply of drugs became apparent in the 1940s, it was the inability to deal with script doctors that remained the principal problem for the Home Office as the 1950s and 1960s ushered in the growth of the London opiate subculture, supported by a range of new prescribing doctors. By the 1950s, script doctors were aware that under the present laws, providing they kept within certain bounds—consisting mainly of adherence to record-keeping requirements—they could not be prosecuted nor their prescribing otherwise curtailed. The number of these practitioners had grown, and the quantities of drugs that could be supplied to addict patients were now in principle virtually unlimited.

Amongst the most notorious of this wave of script doctors was Dr Joseph Rourke of Kensington, perhaps the most prolific of prescribers since the wartime exploits of Dr Quinlan, and whose patients included at one time or another most of the core subcultural addicts in London. Rourke was continually on the Drugs Branch radar between 1953 and his death in 1960. His prescribing was such that, according to the Met, Rourke 'has come to be regarded by that Department (i.e. the Home Office) as the worst "script doctor" ever known to them'.[23] In 1955 Dr Rourke was prosecuted following the death by overdose of one of his West End patients, a Nigerian jazz musician named Broderick Walker.[24] The crux of the prosecution case was that Rourke had aided and abetted Walker to be in unauthorised possession of heroin, which he had simultaneously

[23] TNA MEPO 3/2579, CID Memorandum 9 August 1956.

[24] TNA MH 58/565, Home Office Appendix Case 1 Dr J.M.R.

received from a second practitioner. The prosecution, always misguided, was unsuccessful: the magistrate, Mr Raphael, observed that 'there is nothing in these regulations, to which my attention has been directed, which limits the quantities of drugs that may be lawfully prescribed by a doctor…'.[25] The magistrate observed that the discretion of the doctor to provide the dose he considered appropriate was 'absolute'; Rourke left Marylebone Magistrates' Court with his character unblemished.

The difficulty of intervening to curb the prescribing of these practitioners, then, was still causing the Home Office and Metropolitan Police immense frustrations by the middle years of the 1950s and was apparently what prompted the initiation of the first Brain Report, albeit by a highly circuitous route. By this time, the two dominant sources of concern for the authorities were Rourke and a Clapham-based practitioner who had qualified in 1941: Dr Harry Freeman of Clapham Road.[26]

Opiate Subcultures and Transitions

In general terms, we can summarise the opiate subculture that formed at the beginning of the 1930s as being composed of those from the aristocratic and upper middle classes. Furthermore, there was a strong linkage of this subculture with a particular kind of modern woman: young, often Sapphic or bisexual in her erotic inclinations, modernist by temperament and consequently individualistic and insubordinate toward convention. These young women were the representative figures of the subculture in the press and the law courts and the anxieties of the governing classes.

The 1950s subculture shared a number of characteristics with its precursor; again, it was predominantly young in composition, it regarded itself as modern, and it was sometimes, though less often, accompanied by sexual experimentation. It also arrived as part of a lifestyle associated with American jazz, albeit a different incarnation of jazz. Moreover, both of these subcultural waves appeared shortly after a global war. However, the 1950s subculture's espousal of bohemian attitudes was much less tightly linked with the discourses of the feminine cultural vanguard of the 1930s;

[25] Anon, *British Medical Journal* 2,4942 (1955) p. 797. See also *Times* 9 September 1955, p. 5, and *Daily Mirror* 9 September 1955, p. 5. As to the double-scripting aspects of the case, Rourke had sidestepped potential problems by forging a partnership with Dr Maguire, so they were able to cover each other's patients.

[26] We will hear more of Dr Freeman below.

indeed, it was largely a subculture of young males in which women occupied a subaltern position. In Britain, it was also largely white, despite the presence of six Nigerians in Spear's list of Mark's infected contacts.

One of the addicts on Spear's inventory was Barry Ellis, born in middle-class Surrey in 1926. According to his autobiography, the luridly titled *I Came Back from Hell*, Ellis was introduced to the use of opiates by a tank transporter crew during the intense fighting that followed the Normandy landings.[27] He employed Omnopon to alleviate the trauma of battle and was reintroduced to opiates in 1946 through a chance encounter with Angela Wyndham-Wilson, a 'society addict' in receipt of supplies from Dr Marks Ripka. Ripka was a Gower Street script doctor well known to the Drugs Branch and had also numbered among his patients Brian Dean Paul.[28] Mrs Wyndham-Wilson appeared in court in 1953 accused of unlawful possession of heroin, flanked by two nuns from Spelthorne St Mary's where she was undergoing a cure. She had been involved with a Maltese addict, Joseph Peralta, and her marriage to a British naval officer had broken down.[29]

Ellis' addict career was initiated at the beginning of the end of the classical age of the British System. Interviewed by Marek Kohn in 1990, he described the addict lifestyle of wealthy Wyndham-Wilson, whose bed and Mayfair apartment he had shared briefly in the late 1940s: 'You picked the phone up, you phoned a cab, you phoned a doctor, you phoned a chemist; you didn't even have to move out of bed and the stuff could be brought to your flat half an hour later without you moving.'[30] This was reminiscent of the elite addict lifestyle that Brenda Dean Paul and Anthea Carew had enjoyed in the 1930s; by the time Wyndham-Wilson appeared in court, it was fast disappearing, belonging as it did to a world that was already becoming remote from the jazz cellars and cafes haunted by Dancing Mark and his hipster customers. For a while, Ellis managed to maintain a foot in both camps. Though he was, according to Kohn, never really part of the jazz or beat movement of the 1950s, Ellis was a charismatic figure enjoying enhanced social status amongst the new heroin wave due to his connections with the 1930s subculture and carried 'all my worldly goods…

[27] B. Ellis & A. Revie, *I Came Back From Hell: The story of Barry Ellis* (London: Brown, Watson, 1963) pp. 18–20.

[28] TNA MEPO 3/1054, 'Supplies of large quantities of morphine by Dr. M.D. Ripka to Brian Dean Paul, drug addict, and brother of Brenda Dean Paul, 1936–1947.'

[29] *Daily Express* 12 February 1953, p. 5.; *Daily Telegraph* 12 February 1953, p. 9.

[30] M. Kohn, 'Life and Times: Grains of Truth' *The Guardian*, 1 September 1990.

in a small crocodile holdall, which I inherited from the late Brenda Dean Paul, queen of the junkies'.[31,32] The 'crocodile holdall' was a sacred relic for Ellis, a signifier of subcultural membership.

Subcultural Geography and the West End

In cultural geography, the interwoven fabrics of space, place and culture are analysed.[33] Adding a historical understanding enables one to explore the sediments of meaning laid down, layer upon layer, through the passage of time. In his historical account of heroin use in American cities, urban historian Eric Schneider observes that, 'A drug subculture is rooted in physical spaces that sustain it and allow it to flourish and continue over time.'[34] Schneider's argument is made in the context of his analysis of the postwar expansion of heroin use in New York, a new drug scene which invested spaces that had formerly hosted a marijuana subculture. However, the point that there is a significant spatial dimension to subcultural transmission is a general one and holds good in the case of the development of opiate subcultures in London.

It was in the interlinked spaces of nightclubs, bars, hotels, restaurants, doctors' consulting rooms and pharmacies of London's West End, in addition to certain groups of flats and houses in Mayfair and Chelsea, that the 1930s opiates subculture developed. A similar spatiality was involved in the years following the Second World War as a new wave of heroin subculture emerged; once again, the Soho clubs and cafes played a key role,

[31] Ibid.

[32] Barry Ellis and Alastair Revie, *I Came Back from Hell*, p. 68. As in the case of the published drug narrative of 'Raymond Thorpe', which was ghosted by Derek Agnew (see below), Ellis' biography was co-written with Alastair Revie. Revie and Agnew were tabloid journalists who produced 'social problem' paperbacks, and their moralistic outlook on drugs is deeply interwoven with the recollections of their respective addict co-authors. Thus Ellis' undoubted knowledge of some of the individuals on the heroin scene is supplemented by fantasy, such as his preposterous claim to have been helicoptered to France to meet Charles Luciano, the Italian-American organised crime boss, who wanted to begin trafficking in England. According to Ellis, Brian Howard and his lover Sam Langford were employed as dealers by Luciano. Ellis says he approached Inspector Robert Fabian about this plot, but Fabian, perhaps unsurprisingly, gave little credence to his story.

[33] See, for example, T. S. Oakes, & P. L. Price (eds), *The Cultural Geography Reader* (Abingdon: Routledge, 2008).

[34] E. C. Schneider, (2008) Smack*: Heroin and the American City* (Philadelphia: University of Pennsylvania Press, 2008) p. 17.

alongside a new list of prescribing doctors and the same late-night pharmacies—Boots of Piccadilly and John Bell and Croyden of Wigmore Street. As before, these venues, in combination with flats and rooms, provided locations in which networks of older and more experienced users equipped with practical drug knowledge and drug legends mixed with neophytes, and these modes of knowledge and practices were transmitted to a new generation.

Many of the spaces with which the postwar heroin subculture was associated existed in the same physical locations as their predecessors of the 1920s and 1930s. The best example of this tightly bounded superimposition of historical layers was in the Archer Street area of Soho, near Piccadilly Circus; it is an area centred specifically in and around Ham Yard, just north of the Windmill Theatre at the intersection of Archer Street and Great Windmill Street. In the 1930s, Ham Yard was the location of venues such as the Blue Lantern and the Hambone, both well-known nightclubs frequented by bohemian and literary circles. The Blue Lantern, in particular, was a venue with links to the nascent opiate subculture at the beginning of the 1930s. By the late 1940s, a new wave of jazz music and associated elements of lifestyle and discourse had reached London from New York. Known as 'bebop', it was a modernist jazz form that stood in sharp contrast to the revivalist, traditional or 'trad' jazz, the New Orleans-inspired strand of the genre.[35] Amongst the menu of cultural elements that went to make up the bebop lifestyle was the practice of drug use.

Club Eleven, Modern Jazz and Subcultural Transmission

A number of British modern jazz musicians travelled to New York to see their musical inspirations perform live; as a consequence of the paucity of British venues where bebop could be performed in the immediate postwar years, these musicians lacked money but were able to work their passage by playing in the restaurants and bars of transatlantic liners, bringing back with them to London the musical influences, the recordings and the attitudes toward drugs (cannabis and, especially, cocaine and heroin) of Charlie Parker, Dizzy Gillespie, Miles Davis and others. The core of these

[35] P. Bailey, (2009) 'Jazz at the Spirella: coming of age in Coventry in the 1950s', in B. Conekin, F. Mort & C. Waters (eds) *Moments of Modernity: Reconstructing Britain 1945–1964* (London & New York: Rivers Oram Press, 1999).

British bebop musicians formed the cooperative known as Club Eleven in late 1948.[36] The club's location was significant; situated at Mac's Rehearsal Rooms, Great Windmill Street, it was a minute's walk from the musician's union headquarters in Archer Street. The Harmony Inn on Archer Street was a (very) late-night 'Greasy Spoon' cafe frequented by jazz musicians and Soho criminals; it was here that the bebop players would gather to talk and smoke, and to which their audiences retired after the venues closed. It was in these liminal night-time spaces that the elements making up the early postwar heroin culture came together. According to Raymond Thorpe, who experienced both the clubs and the drug scene of these years, and whose biography was ghosted by tabloid journalist Derek Agnew: 'In the Club Eleven at least one pusher was always hanging around. If you could not find him there it was a certainty someone would be standing on the corner of Archer Street or sitting in the Harmony Inn waiting for business.'[37] There is substantial support for the accuracy of these claims.[38]

The well-known police raid on Club Eleven took place on April 15, 1950, soon after the club had moved to larger premises in nearby Carnaby Street. It resulted in several prosecutions, mostly for cannabis or cocaine, each in small quantities.[39] Before passing sentence, the magistrate at Marlborough Street, who had to have the term 'bebop' explained to him by police officers, commented that 'This sounds a very queer place to me – a very rum place.'[40]

Melody Maker quoted an RAF servicewoman arrested on the night, who declared that the evening 'left me filled with resentment of the police, because I was accused of possessing a low moral standard, fraternising with "buck niggers", and the likelihood of becoming a drug addict', a comment that tells us much about police perceptions of the venue, which

[36] K. Grime, *Jazz at Ronnie Scott's* (London: Robert Hale, 1979).

[37] R. Thorpe & D. Agnew, Viper*: The Confessions of a Drug Addict* (London: Robert Hale, 1956) p. 44.

[38] Anthony John Curtis was a hemp user who later turned to heroin and was believed by the Drugs Branch to represent 'the first recorded instance in the United Kingdom of an adolescent regularly smoking hemp' following his two arrests in 1952. He claimed he had been smoking regularly since he was 16 years of age and was 18 years old at his arrest. Following his placement on probation in August 1952, Curtis was rearrested in October in possession of several small packs of the drug when police raided the Harmony Inn. He was 'sentenced to a period of Borstal training'. TNA MEPO 3/2954, 'UK Annual Report to the United Nations, 1953'.

[39] TNA MEPO 3/2954, *Annual Reports of Governments* UK, 1950.

[40] *The Gloucester Citizen* 15 April 1950, p. 1.

was shut down shortly afterwards, and wider public attitudes toward race and subculture.[41] However, what is of most significance for the present research is not the raid itself but rather the background drug use of the club's founders and their circle. While many (such as Ronnie Scott) consumed drugs on an occasional basis, there were other bebop artistes who were heroin and cocaine users by vocation. Perhaps foremost amongst these was Tommy Pollard, a highly respected pianist and arranger whose heroin use increasingly collided with his responsibilities as a band member. Pollard was a part of the original Club Eleven cooperative but had connections deep in the criminal underworld of Soho and was rumoured to use his expert fast driving skills as a getaway driver in the service of armed robbers. Sometimes regarded as Britain's first high-profile jazz drug fatality, Pollard died in 1960 after several years of ill health and obscurity.[42] Other musicians at the top of the British bebop scene were also dedicated consumers of these drugs, including Phil Seamen, Red Reece, Dickie Devere, Jimmy Deuchar, Tubby Hayes, Stan Tracey, Alan Branscombe and others.

This roster of gifted musicians played a vital role in the diffusion of heroin and cocaine use to their audiences and hangers-on in the club scene. These musicians were drawn to heroin because many of the American jazz greats whom they emulated used the drug and were immersed in its mythology and atmosphere. Younger players often felt that drug use was a necessary passport to insider status in the bebop subculture and a badge of modernity. In addition, heroin insulated the players from the distractions of the outside world, assisting their concentration on the complex instrumental styles that characterised the genre; in more general terms, it enabled a focus to be maintained on 'authentic' subjectivity and kept at an appropriate distance the inauthentic demands of 'square' social life.[43] The influence of Sartre is visible here, albeit refracted through American culture, and would continue to resonate through the attitudes of the new heroin subculture across the 1950s and early 1960s. It was one facet of the continuing relevance of Paris to subcultural developments in London.

[41] Quoted in D. Sandbrook, (2006) *Never Had It So Good: A History of Britain from Suez to the Beatles* (London: Brown, Little, 2006) p. 480.

[42] D. Taylor, http://henrybebop.co.uk/devere2.htmAccessed 18 August 2015.

[43] H. Becker, *Outsiders: Studies in the Sociology of Deviance* (New York: Simon & Schuster, 1997). Becker's well-known work on US musicians and marijuana users offers a number of parallels.

Dickie Devere: Subcultural Transmitter

Certain individuals within the jazz and nightlife milieu played a seminal role in linking the remnants of the 1930s network with the new subculture that took hold in the 1950s. This linkage was forged through social connections in which drug knowledge and charisma accumulated by the older addicts was transmitted to a younger group ready and willing to receive it. Practical know-how included information about, and introduction to, script doctors who could be relied upon to prescribe without too much fuss. It included knowledge of the location of all-night pharmacies, and insider knowledge regarding, for example, the possibility of cashing the next day's prescription at midnight; the practice of double-scripting, including use of aliases, pharmacies to be avoided and so on; who to approach to buy or borrow drugs; illicit sources, including the periodic availability of stolen or imported drugs; how to prepare and to inject one's dose and to minimise withdrawal symptoms; the identification of plain-clothes detectives, places to avoid because of police surveillance and so on. At or near the top of this expanding ladder of forbidden learning was the granting of access to the home of an experienced user, where such forms of illicit pedagogy could be practised at leisure. In short, the proliferation of new heroin networks in the 1950s depended on the flows of drugs and drug knowledge that passed between initiates and neophytes.

Dickie Devere was one of those granted trusted access to the home of Brenda Dean Paul. It was within this inaccessible space that the Drugs Branch—particularly Len Dyke, for whom 'every new addict was a personal defeat'—believed that the core practices of narcotic pedagogy took place.[44,45] During a period of police surveillance in 1956, Devere was listed as one of the regular visitors to the flat occupied by Paul at 28 Sloane Gardens, Chelsea. From here, according to an anonymous informer who had telephoned Dyke at the Drugs Branch in May 1956, Paul supplied retail quantities of cocaine and heroin to visitors to the flat. She had since 1951 been a patient of Dr Harry Freeman, a doctor based in Clapham who provided her with NHS drug treatment. Described by the Home Office as a 'comparatively young and inexperienced doctor', Freeman prescribed Paul 210 grains of cocaine (just under a half an ounce) and 17.5

[44] 'Journal interview 20: Conversation with H. B. Spear' *British Journal of Addiction* 83 (1988) pp. 473–482.

[45] TNA MEPO 3/2579, 'Suspected drug trafficking' Home Office memorandum 30 May 1956.

grains of morphine (just over one gramme) every four days.[46] The cocaine dose was described by Dyke as 'fantastic'. He observed that cocaine, or 'China' as it was then known on the streets of West London, was becoming 'exceedingly fashionable among a circle of addicts already "on" morphine or heroin'.[47] He also claims that the relationship between Paul and Freeman was 'more than doctor-cum-patient', although the police had no knowledge of this alleged involvement.[48,49] Dyke's memorandum reproduces his conversation with the informant and describes Freeman's treatment of Paul as 'one of the worst cases of over-prescribing of drugs by a doctor to a known addict that has ever come to the notice of these authorities'. With Paul receiving almost a half-ounce of pure, pharmaceutical-grade cocaine every few days, Drugs Branch claims that she was selling some of this on, as well as swapping it for heroin and for shoplifted goods such as clothes, do appear plausible. Additionally, it is likely the heroin obtained in this way was sold on to her circle of visitors, given Paul's preference for morphine for her personal consumption.[50]

In addition to being a regular customer with access to the supplies she dealt from her home, Devere was introduced by Brenda to Dr Rourke. Devere was well established within Paul's set; simultaneously, he was a key member of the new group of bebop jazz musicians using heroin and cocaine. These factors placed him in a strong position to operate as a subcultural transmitter, passing on drug know-how and discourse between the two groups. In the early 1950s, Devere was regarded as the best drummer on the British modern jazz scene and provided musical tuition to other celebrated jazz drummers such as Phil Seamen and Red Reece. It is highly likely that he also transmitted drug knowledge, and possibly drugs, to each of them. Both went on to a long-term heroin career.

The mythology that attached itself to heroin use continued to circulate through this network of high-profile musicians and jazz aficionados, radiating outwards together with the practical drug know-how that they possessed. And so the practice of consuming heroin and cocaine proliferated, not through 'infection'—an extended metaphor deployed in governmental,

[46] TNA MEPO 3/2579, CID Memorandum 13 August 1957.

[47] TNA MEPO 3/257 9, 'Suspected drug trafficking' Home Office memorandum 30 May 1956.

[48] Ibid.

[49] TNA MEPO 3/2579, CID Memorandum 9 August 1956.

[50] TNA MEPO 3/2579, 'Suspected drug trafficking' Home Office memorandum 30 May 1956.

clinical and regulatory discourse whose use developed along with an attempt to impose a respectable order on the subculture—but through processes of social and cultural power, pleasure and exchange.

As is usually the case, the perspectives of those using drugs within a host culture hostile to dissidence are hard to obtain. We saw that in similar circumstances in the 1930s, an anonymous postcard represented one of the best opportunities to express some of the discourses circulating in the opiate-using subculture. In the 1950s, a similar opening was created by recourse to the speech of a fictional character, a mouthpiece who provides one of the few surviving accounts of the ways in which the older generation of addicts was viewed by the new wave. Among the participants and most perceptive chroniclers of the early postwar cannabis scene was the novelist Terry Taylor, who was present in London in the 1950s and writes of a fictionalised addict named Popper, who receives a heroin script from one 'Lady Devalera', an obvious alias for Lady Frankau, the 'overprescribing' Wimpole Street psychiatrist at the heart of the conclusions of the second Brain Committee's report.[51] In the novel, Popper has written a poem celebrating the life and death of 'Brenda', an obvious reference to Brenda Dean Paul who had died in 1959 while the book was being written:

> 'Brenda is dead!
> She is no more.
> A 1,000,000,000 pops away
> perched upon a crooked star
> chained to the earth by
> too many memories.
> Is She a Bishop yet?
> Stopped by an acre of hypoforest
> a snowstorm of Snow
> trapped by…'[52]

The poem is read without comprehension by the two cannabis smokers who stumble across it in Popper's notebook, but it is clearly an indication of Taylor's recollection of the ways in which Paul was viewed by the new wave addicts of the period, amongst whom she enjoyed a legendary status.

[51] T. Taylor *Baron's Court All Change. Introduction by Stewart Home* (London: New London Editions, 2011) (First published 1961) p. 97.

[52] Ibid. p. 139.

Other Influences: The USA and France

Alongside the governmental and diplomatic influences that bore upon countries' drug policies, they were affected by discourses and practices emerging from the cultural and social domain. The literary and cultural movement known as 'beat' was an American phenomenon that appeared in the immediate postwar years. It possessed no unified ideology, though it borrowed from both French existentialism and Eastern religions, and valorised individuality, spontaneity and the spirituality of the mundane. Along with these came a fascination with the social outsider and the deviant, and an enthusiasm for sexual and narcotic experimentation. Its literary originators and prominent figures included the poet Allen Ginsberg and the novelists Jack Kerouac and John Clellon Holmes. William Burroughs is usually classified as a beat writer, and there were several other important figures involved. In Britain, Alexander Trocchi and Colin MacInnes, in addition to Taylor, were the main writers working within the genre.

Judith Blackwell is right to point to the importance of the American beat discourse to the growth of the postwar London heroin subculture; however, the influence of France was also important. The existentialist movement was in some ways a parallel to what was happening in America, though it is often associated with the work of Sartre, who looked to the novel to express his perspectives on the contemporary world, as did Camus and others. Moreover, popular existentialism was deeply linked to a specific stylistic and aesthetic cluster: philosopher Jonathon Webber has called it 'the existentialism of black clothes and jazz clubs, coffee and cigarettes'.[53] In parts of bohemian London, including Chelsea and Soho, this cluster of objects and meanings included heroin.

Just as it had in the 1930s, postwar Paris acted as a magnet for the young Americans of the 1950s, and a similar pattern of connections existed with regard to drugs. The Scottish beat novelist Alex Trocchi had been introduced to opiates by Jean Cocteau in Paris.[54] Moreover, it was not merely famous literary figures whose drug habits could be traced to Parisian networking. The *Daily Express* had been one of several newspapers running serialised pieces on the growing London drug scene, and inserted into this narrative the case of Christine Vasey, who was arrested at

[53] J. Webber, 'Existentialism' in J. Skorupski (ed), *Routledge Companion to Ethics* (London: Routledge, 2012) pp. 230–240.

[54] A. Campbell & T. Niel (eds) *A Life in Pieces: Reflections on Alexander Trocchi* (Edinburgh: Rebel Inc., 1997) p. 152.

Northolt Airport in August 1951 with Indian hemp, heroin and a syringe in her handbag. The drugs had allegedly been obtained at 'wild bohemian parties' in the French capital. The *Express* made much of a customs officer's warning that 'Indian Hemp is the first stage on the downward path', leading on to heroin. DS Lyle was present in court to testify that Vasey had been 'mixing with traffickers and drug addicts for the past six months'.[55]

Paris was the major European hub for American jazz musicians, though by the early 1960s the trafficking of heroin sometimes flowed in the opposite direction from that of the 1930s, with London becoming a source of supply for some of Paris' young cosmopolitan drug consumers. The American jazz singer and trumpet player Chet Baker, living in Paris and enjoying considerable fame at this time, spoke in his memoirs of crossing the channel to visit Lady Frankau's London consulting rooms, she having established a global reputation for the ready availability of generous prescriptions for heroin and cocaine. Baker wrote: 'On our first day in England…I went to 32 Wimpole Street to see Lady Isabelle MacDougall Frankau…She didn't ask me for much information about myself…She simply asked for my name, my address, and how much cocaine or heroin I wanted per day.'[56] The Drugs Branch was alarmed by public announcements of the ease with which Baker had acquired heroin under the auspices of the British System. 'I worked in Paris for a while, then came to England, knowing that drugs were fairly easy to obtain. But the degree of facility opened my eyes', he told the publication *Today*.[57] Another, unnamed American addict told Metropolitan Police officers that 'it was common knowledge among drug addicts in Paris that drugs were easily obtained through this doctor (Lady Frankau)…'.[58]

Regulatory Responses: The International Domain

The regulatory shifts in the postwar era have been attributed by researchers such as Smart or Bing Spear as stemming from international factors; others, such as Stimson and Oppenheimer, saw them as a response to the

[55] *Daily Express* 07 March 1952, p. 3.

[56] C. Baker, *As Though I Had Wings: The Lost Memoir* (London: Indigo, 1997) p. 97.

[57] TNA HO 319/2, Home Office Annex: 'Cases of foreign addicts attracted to this country'.

[58] Ibid.

growth of domestic drug use.[59] In fact, the two levels of drug control are tightly interwoven, and each played a part in the changes that overtook the regulatory order in the 1950s and 1960s. The international dimension was always important, but in the period preceding the agreement of the 1961 Single Convention, it was especially significant as countries sought to shape the draft treaty to suit their national interests.[60]

Following the war and the rise of the USA as an international military, political and economic superpower, there was friction between it and Britain over aspects of the latter's drug policies. The 1955 American attempt to impose a global prohibition on heroin was eventually faced down by the British government after pressure from the medical profession in support of the drug's retention in medical treatment.[61] Britain's representative at the Commission on Narcotic Drugs (CND), the policy-making body for the new UN international drug control system, was J. H. 'Johnny' Walker. Spear identifies Walker as providing the initiative that led to the first Brain Committee, which, commencing its meetings in 1958, reviewed the British System of drug control for the first time since Rolleston.[62] Government documentation from the mid- to late 1950s supports the claim.[63] The context for Walker's views was largely international, with the British System undergoing criticism from a number of countries, particularly the USA, through the mechanism of the new United Nations drug control regime.[64]

In 1955, Walker sent a lengthy and thoughtful memorandum to the Home Office suggesting that it was time to look again at the British drug control system. Despite the system's smooth domestic running, said Walker: 'It so happens that a number of problems have arisen, or are on the horizon, which indicate that this is a suitable moment to review the present system of control.'[65] These problems or potential problems

[59] C. Smart, 'Social Policy and Drug Dependence: An Historical Case Study' Drug *and Alcohol Dependence* 16 (1985) pp. 169–180; Spear, H. B. *Heroin Addiction, Care and Control*, pp. 90–95; G. V. Stimson & E. Oppenheimer *Heroin Addiction: Treatment and control in Britain* (London: Tavistock, 1982) p. 40.

[60] D. R. Bewley-Taylor, The *United States and International Drug Control, 1909–1997* (London and New York: Continuum, 1999) p. 141.

[61] H. B. Spear, *Heroin Addiction, Care and Control* pp. 65–89.

[62] Spear, H.B., *Heroin Addiction, Care and Control* p. 90.

[63] TNA HO 319/1 and MH 58/565.

[64] D. R. Bewley-Taylor, *The United States and International Drug Control, 1909–1997* (London: Continuum, 1999).

[65] TNA HO 319/1 'Dangerous Drugs Administration and Policy in the United Kingdom' 25 October 1955.

included the proliferation of new synthetic drugs such as pethidine and methadone, the UK policy on addiction (by which was meant in particular the Rolleston-inspired regulations permitting the long term of maintenance of opiate habits and the belief in the 'stabilised addict'), addict doctors and improper prescribing and supplies to addicts (the issues surrounding script doctors). The memorandum paid the greatest attention to the second and the fourth of these categories, replicating the situation that obtained when the Rolleston Committee reported and showing that the issue of doctors prescribing dangerous drugs to addicts had remained at the heart of governmental anxieties. Walker claimed that the Rolleston Committee never intended the 'lavish supply of dangerous drugs to addicts merely for the maintenance of addiction'.[66] He then made reference to a 'small but potentially dangerous group of drug addicts (mainly heroin addicts) in London at the present time'.[67] This group was 'disturbing', as it represented 'the first real sign of a significant increase in heroin addiction for very many years'.[68] The group's members had become addicted young and were mostly under 30—often nearer 20; many shared an involvement in one particular field of entertainment and therefore met socially at regular intervals—a reference to the jazz club scene. The social context of this drug use made it ripe for proselytism, contended Walker, 'always one of the more dangerous features of drug addiction'.

He continued that many 'appear to obtain supplies from a small number of doctors who make no attempt whatever at cure or even, so far as can be judged, at reduction of the dose. In other words, their addiction is deliberately fed, almost certainly in some instances for purposes of gain'.[69] Walker concluded that: 'The "script doctor" who thus makes drugs freely available to addicts represents a special problem….'[70]

Walker's memorandum showed that the Home Office was by this time fully aware of the flourishing new London addict subculture, a full ten years before these facts were published in the second Brain Report. As noted by Spear, the peculiar thing is that the first Brain Committee did not address it in their deliberations nor their report.[71] At the Home Office, it was Tom Green (who succeeded Walker at the Drugs Branch) who led the

[66] Ibid.
[67] Ibid.
[68] Ibid.
[69] Ibid.
[70] Ibid.
[71] Spear, H. B., *Heroin Addiction, Care and Control*, p. 92.

drafting of the advice and information sent to the Ministry of Health, from which emerged the shape of the review. For 'some inexplicable reason', while drawing heavily on Walker, Green did not include evidence of the emergence of London's expanding heroin subculture.[72]

One possible reason for this startling omission lay in the international relations around the topic of drug control. Walker points out that US medical opinion was firmly against maintenance and the notion of the stable addict. The strongly held view in the American medical profession was that it is ethically unacceptable to condemn a patient, especially a young patient, to perpetual addiction by offering this form of treatment. It was also remarked that the CND and World Health Organization were highly critical of ambulatory treatment of the kind practised in the UK. Indeed at its tenth session, the CND 'expressed the view that ambulatory treatment (including the so-called "clinic" method) was not advisable and asked the World Health Organization to prepare a study on the appropriate methods of treatment'.[73] Furthermore, a clause had recently been inserted into the draft Single Convention which spoke of treatment being given on 'a planned and compulsory basis, in properly conducted and duly authorised institutions'.[74,75] However, by virtue of a qualifying clause that was initiated by the UK, such measures would be applicable only in those countries having a large addict population; it was this proviso that permitted the UK government to sign the 1961 treaty despite its differences with respect to drug treatment. Notwithstanding this, Walker expressed concern that the general trend at the CND was toward compulsion and that there may in due course be concerted pressure for the removal of the UK clause. He added that 'it is unlikely that the United Kingdom could ever accept an obligation to require compulsory treatment of drug addicts in a closed institution'.[76] In fact, Walker made it clear

[72] Ibid.

[73] The Tenth Session of the Commission on Narcotic Drugs, 1955. http://www.unodc.org/unodc/en/data-and-analysis/bulletin/bulletin_1955-01-01_2_page005.html Accessed 3rd September 2013.

[74] The Single Convention was the proposed new UN treaty to restructure and harmonise previously existing international drug control law. It was adopted by plenipotentiary conference in 1961 and still forms the foundations of the present international drug control regime.

[75] TNA HO 319/1, 'Dangerous Drugs Administration and Policy in the United Kingdom' 25 October 1955. In this passage, Walker was quoting from a 1954 CND draft of the Single Convention.

[76] Ibid.

that such a measure could prevent the UK from signing the treaty, and would have been in conflict with the overall trend of mental health policies in Britain at this time, as expressed in Lord Percy's 1957 *Report of the Royal Commission on the Law Relating to Mental Illness and Mental Deficiency*.[77] This optimistic document led the trend away from confinement, toward voluntary and community-based mental health treatment, and fed into the 1959 Mental Health Act. In relation to addiction, Walker commented in closing that: 'There is a limit to what the State should attempt, and the deprivation of personal liberty for medical reasons is far too serious a matter to contemplate unless there is overwhelming evidence of the need for it because of some widespread and particularly virulent social problem. This need does not exist in the United Kingdom.'

This last sentence is the key one. In order to fight its corner at the CND, the UK government needed powerful evidence that the domestic drug problem continued to be so small as to be negligible, a point which some other countries disputed. Consequently, 'there would be much to be said from the point of view of strengthening our case in international circles for obtaining an authoritative opinion from a body of experts on the necessity for, and the feasibility of, providing special treatment for drug addicts in this country'.[78] In other words, a committee set up to review Britain's arrangements could prove very useful in providing the government with ammunition to fight its international drug policy corner, so long as this evidence indicated that the problem was tiny and relatively insignificant.

Although, as Spear claims, Walker's superiors at the Home Office were initially unreceptive to his argument, it may well have been influential at the meetings of the Brain Committee, which produced the first report. Green led the way in producing the documentation for the Committee; mention of the expansion of the opiate subculture was entirely absent, and the growth in heroin addiction strongly downplayed. Accordingly, its report was structured on precisely the lines that would support the government in its negotiations at the CND. It stated baldly: 'After careful examination of all the data put before us we are of the opinion that in Great Britain the incidence of addiction to dangerous drugs… is still very small.'[79]

[77] E. Percy Baron of Newcastle *Report of the Royal Commission on the Law relating to Mental Illness and Mental Deficiency* (London: HMSO, 1957).

[78] Ibid.

[79] *Report of the Interdepartmental Committee on Drug Addiction* 1961 London: HMSO. Paragraph 24.

This argument remains for the present a speculative one; nonetheless, the omission of the West End heroin subculture from the Home Office memorandum of evidence to the first Brain Committee and the report's conclusion, which supports the UK's requirements at CND in the run-up to the 1961 Single Convention, are highly suggestive.

The Regulatory Response in the Domestic Domain

As we have seen, the Met too was well aware that drug use was increasing in London, beginning with the spread of Indian hemp consumption beyond its customary lodging in the African and Asian immigrant communities and the West End entertainment district. After the Second World War, a small, specialist drug squad was formed by the Metropolitan Police, comprising one detective sergeant (DS) who dealt with drugs inquiries and two more who were available to assist him as required. The three policemen and the senior officer to whom they reported had remained in close contact with the Home Office since the squad's inception in 1947.[80] The lead officer was DS George Lyle, who succeeded Dyke as the drugs expert in the Met. Having moved from his native Scotland to the capital to join the force in 1936, Lyle served in the RAF during the Second World War, returning to police duties following the end of hostilities. During the 1950s, the Metropolitan Police Drugs Office (as it was then known) was increased to 1 DS (first class), 1 DS (second class) and 3 detective constables (DCs), and a major overhaul in the 1960s saw the unit increased to 14 full-time officers headed up by a detective superintendent.[81] It was noted, pointedly, that: 'Over the years there has been a steady increase in the work of the Dangerous Drugs Squad, but this increase has become even more marked since the Commonwealth immigrants arrived in this country in such substantial numbers.'[82]

Though much of the unit's focus was on cannabis, it was at this stage that the Chemist Inspection duties were assigned to this central drug squad, a move of major importance in the policing of opiate addiction and its subculture. Previously, and to the continuous annoyance of the Home Office, these duties had been carried out by officers at local police stations, who had no special expertise in examining dangerous drugs registers and

[80] TNA HO 45/24948, Annual Report of Drugs Branch, 1947.
[81] TNA MEPO 2/10167, C.O.C.1 Memorandum 28 June 1963.
[82] TNA MEPO 2/10167, Dangerous Drugs Office, C.O.C.1 Branch 28 January 1963.

were regularly accused of failing to identify cases of transgressive prescribing and addiction. The officers at the drugs office had concentrated instead on trafficking and illicit consumption. After the war, the Home Office Drugs Branch again noted that the standard of the Met's Chemist Inspection performance was not high, despite the fact that the London area 'covers about a quarter of the country's population including the majority of the "vicious" addicts'.[83] The lack of a centralised full-time staff for the Chemist Inspection work was held responsible for the poor quality of the results. When Thornton and Dyke visited the Met's Detective Training School at Hendon in 1953, Thornton told the senior officer on duty that, 'when considering police reports of suspected irregularities discovered by police visits to chemists, he was concerned with the comparatively few reports received from the Metropolitan Police compared with those received from the rest of the country'.[84]

Dissatisfaction with the Met's performance of their Chemist Inspection duties continued to grow at the Drugs Branch. Finally, concrete action was prompted by a visit to Glasgow made by Spear in 1959, in which the efficiency of the local Glasgow City Police force in these duties proved something of an eye-opener for the Drugs Branch inspector, contrasting as it did with the Met's own efforts. The key factor underlying the differences in performance, judged Spear, was that the Glasgow inspections were carried out by a team of specialist drugs officers with a high degree of expert knowledge; the unit was dedicated solely to drugs work and was used as a resource by colleagues throughout the Glasgow force and by other police forces around the country. Spear was convinced that very few cases of large or extended prescribing of dangerous drugs would have escaped their attention.[85] The situation in the Met was different due to the mode of organisation of its inspections. In London, inspecting officers carried out a wide range of other police duties, and the Branch had formed the impression over many years that, when pressures conflicted, it was the drugs work that was accorded the lowest priority.

Spear's analysis was supported by his superior, Charles Jeffery, who approached the Metropolitan Police with a proposal that the Chemist Inspection work be remodelled along the lines of the Glasgow force.[86]

[83] TNA HO 45/24948, Annual Report of Drugs Branch, 1946.
[84] TNA MEPO 2/9631, Letter to A.C.C. 12 May 1953.
[85] TNA HO 319/5, Memorandum 21 May 1959.
[86] TNA HO 319/5, Jeffery note 26 May 1959.

However, while there was support amongst a number of senior officers at the Met, there was also a generalised and not inconsiderable hostility to the police taking responsibility for the task of retail chemist shop inspection. It was a task which reached back to the early years of the British System, within which police inspections were such an important component.

It would be several years before the suggested changes were made. They were eventually forced upon the Met when the Home Office identified several cases of long-term prescribing for morphine addiction which had gone unnoticed; one involved a patient prescribed continually for 12 years without the fact coming to light in police inspections, another for 9 years. Armed with these facts and the backing of an 'extremely perturbed' secretary of state, the Home Office was able to twist the arm of the Met.

The impact of these shortcomings in police performance was significant for the construction of the Branch's Addicts Index. The Index was the source of the data on which the published annual addiction statistics were based, and the failure of the inspection system in much of London must have led to the underestimation of addicts receiving prescribed supplies. It is impossible now to estimate by how much the totals fell short, but certainly prior to the 1960s, the figures for the London district, the centre of Britain's opiate subculture, were unreliable.

Dyke's Informant

Meanwhile, 'Len' Dyke of the Drugs Branch was mulling over the implications of his interview with an informant who had supplied details of Brenda Dean Paul's sales of cocaine and heroin. The informant had told Dyke that Paul 'is not only being handsomely rewarded in terms of cash but is *creating* addicts, several of whom are not yet attending any doctor for a lawful supply'.[87] Following the failure of the attempt to prosecute Dr Rourke and the magistrate's subsequent remarks concerning the absence of any limit placed on dosages by the dangerous drugs regulations, it was obvious that neither the Home Office nor the Ministry of Health could intervene to curtail the prescribing of Dr Freeman, who was supplying Paul with extremely high levels of cocaine. Dyke concluded that '(a)s the

[87] TNA MEPO 3/2579, 'Memorandum: Brenda Dean Paul: Suspected Drug Trafficking' A. L. Dyke, 30 May 1956.

matter stands it is a criminal one and only the police are competent to handle it, and with this end in view I will confer with N. S. Y. in the hope that some result may be achieved'.[88]

Dyke's memorandum outlining the case was duly submitted to the Met and initially reviewed by Detective Inspector Fensome of Scotland Yard. In consequence, Paul's premises were placed under surveillance, but the geography of the building prevented police from identifying her callers. The four-storey building in Sloane Gardens, Chelsea, was subdivided into flats, with access obtained via an intercom system at the front door. It was impossible for the watching police to ascertain which premises were being visited. On the other hand, if there were known addicts visiting Paul, they could be identified coming and going, but police were then presented with another problem; if they were in receipt of lawful supplies of heroin or cocaine from a doctor, it would often be impossible to tell which quantities were legitimate and which were not.[89]

Fensome also mentioned communications sent to the Home Office by the Met following the failure of the case against Dr Rourke, which raised similar questions. It was suggested by the police that changes be made to the legislation in order to restrict his supplies to addicts, initially by requiring a second medical opinion to be obtained prior to any prescribing and secondly by limiting the amount of time for which an addict could be supplied by a doctor without a hospital-based residential cure being attempted. Shortly thereafter, the Met received a Home Office reply stating that there was little prospect of these measures being introduced.[90]

In the Met's internal discussion of the problem, Fensome now told his superior that:

> it is quite obvious that both the doctors mentioned in this report (i.e. Rourke and Freeman) prescribe the drugs to such of their patients, as are known addicts, for the gratification of addiction, and in direct contravention of the recommendations of the Rolleston Committee. Whilst they are enabled to carry on in their present manner, knowing full well that there is not the slightest chance of them being prosecuted, there is no possibility of the number of addicts they treat dwindling.[91]

[88] Ibid.

[89] TNA MEPO 3/2579, CID Memorandum, D. I. Fensome, 6 July 1956.

[90] TNA MEPO 3/2579, Fensome to Miller, 9 August 1956.

[91] Ibid.

Fensome concluded by stating that unless the nameless informant was prepared to attend court and give a sworn statement, the police too were unable to act on the case. Superintendent Miller added that, 'If this informant has such a vast knowledge of the activities of drug addicts surely, at times, he/she must be in a position to supply Mr Dyke and/or police with such information that could be acted upon with immediate success.'[92] However, no such information was provided.

The Demise of the Classic British System

The Committee under the chairmanship of Russell Brain began sitting in 1958 and published its report in 1961. The Committee's mandate was to review the advice given in the Rolleston Report of 1926; in particular, to explore the need for fresh provisions in relation to the new synthetic drugs that had appeared since that year; to consider the possibility of providing new treatment, including residential forms; to make recommendations to the government, including on administrative questions.

The Committee judged that addiction in the UK remained a numerically insignificant phenomenon and recommended against registration, compulsory treatment, further statutory controls on new drugs and medical tribunals for transgressive practitioners. In general, it remained close to the logic and ethical framework of its 1926 predecessor. At the famous meeting of the Society for the Study of Addiction at which Lord Brain had first publicly outlined his findings prior to their official publication, pharmacist Irving Benjamin, who worked at John Bell and Croyden and knew many of those who cashed their prescriptions there, had embarrassed Russell Brain. The latter had spoken of 'one or two' script doctors (the term was not employed, having been removed from the Committee's draft documents) in the past 20 years, of the illicit supplies of heroin and cocaine being 'negligible', of the numbers of addicts reducing since the 1930s, of which 'nearly all' were known to the Home Office. Benjamin, who attended the meeting in the company of Spear, spoke out to considerable effect. Lord Brain's optimism, he said, had 'amazed' him. It was unreasonable to assume that the Home Office knew of 'nearly all' addicts; and, 'as to the suggestion that there seems to be no large centre of addiction, I personally can record forty or fifty cocaine, heroin and morphine addicts in the London area alone'.[93]

[92] Ibid.

[93] R. Brain, 'The Report of the Interdepartmental Committee on Drug Addiction' British *Journal of Addiction to Alcohol & Other Drugs* 57,2 (1961) pp. 81–103.

The first Brain Report was subject to considerable criticism and the Committee accused of complacency.[94] Addiction continued to grow rapidly, especially with respect to heroin, and the Committee was reconvened in 1964, publishing a second report in the subsequent year. It recommended notification of addicts, the establishment of the clinic system and restriction of the right to supply heroin and cocaine to doctors on the clinic staff. Doctors who contravened the new system should be brought before the disciplinary committee of the GMC. The key element in the regulatory changes stemming from the second Brain Report was the end of ambulatory treatment—an addict could no longer visit their doctor of choice for drug treatment and live freely as a drug consumer.

By the time of the second Brain Report's appearance, the bebop jazz scene had largely burned itself out. The close connection of postwar drug subcultures with youth culture meant that they were driven by fast-moving shifts in fashion, music and popular culture. From this time, the cultural revolution of the 1960s attached itself, by and large, not to opiates but to the counter culture with its preference for cannabis and LSD.[95]

[94] A. S. Trebach, *The Heroin Solution* Second Edition (Bloomington, Indiana: Unlimited Publishing, 2006), p. 102.

[95] M. Donnelly, *Sixties Britain: Culture, Society and Politics* (Harlow: Pearson, 2005) pp. 123–30.

CHAPTER 9

Concluding Themes

White Drug Culture in the 'Quiet Times'

The research on which this book is based has focused on a set of interlinked hypotheses and inquiries regarding the subculture of UK drug consumption and the regulatory architecture that set out to manage and control it. In terms of periodisation, it has concerned itself with what former Home Office Drugs Branch Chief Inspector 'Bing' Spear characterised as the 'quiet times' of the 1920s to the 1950s.[1] It was an episode during which the narcotic landscape of the UK is considered by many researchers to be largely uneventful. The present research, however, was driven by my own hypothesis that the quiet times were considerably more active, dynamic and significant than had previously been believed to be the case. In the process of exploring this domain, the book makes what I hope are several advances to our knowledge of the history of drug use and its regulation in the UK, particularly during the interwar years, which lie at the heart of the work.

A fundamental question at the core of the research concerned the dating of the emergence of the UK opiate subculture. Traditional historiography has this subculture appearing in the postwar years, either the 1950s or the 1960s. It has been widely argued that the morphine and heroin addicts of the interwar years consisted of a medicalised and respectable

[1] H. B. Spear, 'The early years of Britain's drug situation in practice: up to the 1960s' in J. Strang and M. Gossop, (eds) *Heroin Addiction and the British System: Volume 1: Origins and Evolution* (London and New York: Routledge, 2005) p. 20.

C. Hallam, *White Drug Cultures and Regulation in London, 1916–1960*, https://doi.org/10.1007/978-3-319-94770-9_9

population, often viewed as the mirror-image of the 1960s subcultural addicts. However, the archival and textual evidence consulted in the course of the research does not support this argument, either in terms of the periodisation of the subculture or its characteristics. On the contrary, I believe that this book, which consists of an interwoven set of case studies, provides a convincing demonstration that a white drug culture appeared significantly earlier than has been supposed and was present during the early 1930s. At this juncture, elements of the upper-class bohemia shifted from a reliance on alcohol, 'pick-me-ups' and occasional drug use to a lifestyle centred on the consumption of heroin and/or morphine, with cocaine often playing a secondary role. Composed of a network based in Chelsea, this hedonistic subculture was also notable in its rejection of heterosexual norms, and included a high proportion of homosexuals, lesbians and bisexuals. The leading figures in these groups tended to be young women, many of whom came from the elite classes but were *déclassé* due to their expenditure on drugs, their disreputable conduct and their appearances in court cases that were often reported sensationally in the local, national and international press. Much of the evidence regarding the Chelsea sets is derived from Metropolitan Police files stored at the National Archive; the key file, which has been previously inaccessible, deals with Brenda Dean Paul and her associates and was opened through a Freedom of Information application made by the author.[2] This large and very rich file was supplemented by a range of memoirs and biographies, alongside newspapers sourced from online archives. The combination gave a picture of the individuals and sets involved, helping to show how social and cultural linkages assembled the networks that made up the subculture. I conclude that the research which had understood the addicts of the 1930s as the conceptual opposite of the 1960s subcultural addicts was inaccurate.

Around the same time that the Chelsea network crystallised from the bohemian 'bright young people', a second group of subcultural heroin users emerged from the night-time economy of London's West End. Unlike the Chelsea network that sourced its drugs primarily from doctors prescribing under the terms of the 'British System', the West End network arranged to purchase supplies from illicit sources, particularly from its underworld contacts in Paris. The drugs were obtained either by letter or

[2]TNA MEPO 3/2579, 'Brenda Dean Paul, Drug Addict: activities and associates' 1931–1963.

crossing the channel on the boat train from London. Cocaine also circulated in this network, along with Indian hemp or cannabis.[3]

The drug use of both groups was linked to a more generalised sense of marginality from mainstream society and was interwoven with the contemporary debates and disputes between Victorianism and modernism, differing versions of English identity, conservatism and libertarian culture, and questions of sexuality and gender. There was an ongoing conflict between the drug subculture and the structures that sought to restrict it, including the Home Office, the police, elements of the medical profession and the diffuse social monitoring that is here termed the 'lay culture of surveillance'. Consequently, drugs became entangled with the broader conflicts in British social, cultural and political life, playing a symbolic function within these struggles, in which they were felt to signify the health or pathology of individuals and the nation.

The early white drug subculture differed from the heroin which was to exist in the 1960s in the leading role that was played by women. In other ways, the 1930s groups shared many of the subcultural characteristics of the postwar addicts, living a bohemian lifestyle centred on the acquisition and use of drugs and rejecting the mainstream attitudes and routines of the host culture. Moreover, it was notable that these people were not the isolated addicts pictured in psychiatric discourse and postwar historiography. Gregarious and hedonistic, and with little respect for norm or law, they consumed their drugs together in flats and houses, at clubs and parties; even their appearances in court were social occasions, with friends in attendance in the public gallery and dressed up in their fashionable finery.

The Rolleston Model

The development of drug subculture was bound up with the growth of the juridical and medical structures regulations whose objective was to suppress or manage it. These structures ranged from the international treaties administered by the League of Nations to domestic legislation and regulations thereunder. Following the passage of the Dangerous Drugs Act of 1920 and the police intervention it facilitated, the street drug scene diminished, but recourse to doctors and forged prescriptions continued to provide a steady source of supplies. A Departmental Committee was set up

[3] J. H. Mills, *Cannabis Nation: Control and Consumption in Britain, 1928–2008* (Oxford: Oxford University Press, 2012) pp. 20–24.

in 1924 under the chairmanship of Sir Humphrey Rolleston, its objection to review in what circumstances, if any, heroin and morphine should be supplied to addicts. Its 1926 Report was the founding document of what became known as the 'British System', allowing doctors to supply drugs for the medical treatment of addicts.[4]

This book has examined the day-to-day workings of the system devised by the Rolleston Committee, particularly the supply to addicts and the ways in which the doctors involved in providing these supplies were monitored, reviewed and disciplined by state and professional agencies. Doctors collaborated with the Home Office surveillance of prescribing practitioners through the involvement of the Ministry of Health's Regional Medical Officers, who would visit and interview physicians suspected of transgressive prescribing to addicts or of being addicted themselves. Like the police inspection of retail pharmacies, the assessment of fellow professionals was, from its inception, a task that was undertaken grudgingly.

Medical Conflict over Rolleston

The medical profession in general was conflicted in its views toward the Rolleston model. Central to the supply of the opiate subculture were those practitioners known to the Home Office Drugs Branch as 'script doctors', a term that entered into Drugs Branch use in the 1930s. Some observers have contended that these transgressive practitioners emerged in the 1950s along with the new postwar addict subculture. Archival evidence, however, points to their much earlier arrival; the first known transgressive prescriber, who catered to a group of proto-subcultural addicts, appeared before the General Medical Council in 1917. The most prolific of these doctors, Dr Samuel Connor, practised between 1919 and 1926 and possibly earlier.[5] When his authority to supply dangerous drugs was removed by the secretary of state in 1926, he became a regular abortionist. The connection between the supply of drugs and the provision of abortions was a frequent one amongst these practitioners.[6]

[4] *Departmental Committee on Morphine and Heroin Addiction: Report* (London: HMSO, 1926).

[5] TNA MH 58/277, Appendix 1. Case 1. See also, *British Medical Journal* 1,3406, (1926), pp. 677–678.

[6] TNA MEPO 3/1023 'Dr Samuel Graham Connor: systematic treatment of a number of women for the purpose of procuring abortions (sixteen counts) 1937–1942'.

Script doctors provided large doses of heroin, morphine and cocaine and were willing to disregard the regulations under the Dangerous Drugs Acts. They were a powerful influence in maintaining the opiate subculture. The Drugs Branch believed that they were motivated primarily by the fees that addicts were willing to pay; on the other hand, they undoubtedly provided a service that was flexible and responsive and gave the 'patients' what they wanted.

Numerous practitioners viewed the Rolleston model as wholly ineffective, as was demonstrated by the deliberations of the Royal College of Physicians Committee on Addiction in 1938.[7] The Committee was composed mainly of high-profile addiction specialists, many of whom were trained in psychiatry. In addition, there was a powerful eugenic influence amongst the Committee and a belief that it was necessary to change the law in order to confine addicts and compel them to adopt an abstinent lifestyle. Sharing this detention would be homosexuals and alcoholics, who also made up part of the 'deviant nation'. However, the UK government, including most of those representing the Home Office, had little enthusiasm for this eugenic project, and it did not progress beyond the discourse of the RCP Committee.

Policing Dangerous Drugs

The Metropolitan Police formed its drugs office in 1954, and this is often viewed as the first such unit; however—and this is a familiar theme—such events predated those of the customary historical narrative. There were drugs offices and teams in action well before this. Early actions against the drug trade were carried out by ad hoc units reaching back to the First World War and the 1920s, and these were often unconnected with the CIOs who inspected the dangerous drugs registers of retail pharmacies. According to the records of the Home Office Drugs Branch, a small drug squad was set up in London in 1947, doubtless in response to the authorities' anxieties concerning the growth in consumption in the immediate postwar context.

The CIOs provided information regarding supplies of drugs to addicts as a result of their statutory duty to inspect dangerous drugs registers, which gave them close contact with pharmacy records. They were the

[7] Royal College of Physicians: Committee on Drug Addiction. Minutes of Meeting, 18 January 1938.

primary source of data for Home Office submissions to the League of Nations. This statistical evidence was nonetheless extremely patchy, as many inspections were incomplete and inefficient. This was especially the case in London, where most of the vicious addicts lived. Aside from the CIOs, the major police source of intelligence was the informants with whom officers built up relationships. This network of informants was much more efficient in the capital and compensated somewhat for the haphazard inspections of chemist shops.

Morphine and Morale

Another period of drug policy that had not been previously examined by academic researchers was the Second World War. Exploring the response to the war led the research into an often-unexplored territory in drug legislation and policy—the provision of controlled drugs for medical and scientific purposes. The international conventions and the domestic laws that they obliged countries to enact are often understood as solely prohibitive powers; in fact, they are part of a dual imperative, intended to limit the production, distribution and possession of drugs to medical and scientific purposes. In the Second World War, fears that air attacks would degrade civilian morale led doctors and the Ministry of Health to call for the provision of morphine throughout the social body and to lessen restrictive forms of control over powerful analgesic drugs. This led to conflicts between the Ministry of Health and the Home Office, with the latter continuing to favour tough restriction. Ultimately, driven by the exigencies of war, the Home Office shifted to a more pragmatic orientation, loosening controls over morphine in order to protect the population against 'hysteria' and panic in the face of mass air raids.[8]

Meanwhile, the Drugs Branch maintained its vigilance toward vicious addicts and the script doctors that supplied them, and drug consumers were subject to an intensified stigma against the backdrop of the 'People's War'. In this context, the population pulled together, but the addict networks did whatever they could to exploit the enhanced presence of opiates distributed throughout society. Addicts such as Brenda Dean Paul received highly punitive sentences in return for their drug use and their continued inhabitation of the outsider status.

[8] HO 45/21172 'Relaxation of regulations to allow administration of morphine by approved persons in war emergency conditions. Control and storage of drugs at wartime first aid posts and in factories under government administration.' (1938–1947).

Postwar Developments

The advent of the postwar drug subculture did not sprout from nowhere or result solely from cultural developments in the USA. Undoubtedly, the influence of American and some aspects of French culture was considerable; however, it was combined with subcultural transmissions, within the UK, from the older, interwar addict scene, which included practical drug knowledge. Information regarding script doctors, which could include introductions and references to compliant doctors; injection and other techniques for consumption; people and places from drugs could be obtained—all these and more were transmitted from the older addicts to the novices. There were key individuals that played such roles of subcultural transition and transmission, some of them jazz musicians and writers, who moved across and between interwar and postwar networks.

Last Word

Those who have studied London's homosexual networks, such as Frank Mort, have had remarkably little to say concerning the question of drugs. Admittedly, Mort's focus is on queer communities, and he may reasonably claim that drugs are outside his remit. Nonetheless, historical evidence strongly suggests a high degree of overlap between various bohemian and subcultural groups, with the Chelsea network, for example, demonstrating powerful linkages across drug-using and homosexual/Sapphic networks. Historians of queer experience and social life would surely benefit from breaking down the ghetto that continues to surround drugs, in an age when the cultural conversation on drugs is undergoing profound shifts.

These superimposed bohemias and subcultures link, in turn, to issues of place and space. It is noteworthy that the same locations continue to be associated with drug use over decades. While Soho has been the object of recent historical research, previous scholars have done little to examine London zones such as Chelsea and Mayfair.[9] This is likely to be a result of the focus on working-class drug use, while, in fact, elite groups have played an important role in initiating the UK's drug subculture.

[9] See Slater, S. *Street sex for sale in Soho 1918–39: Experiences, Representation and Attempts at Control.* Unpublished PhD Thesis, University of London, 2007; and, Walkowitz, J. R. *Nights Out: Life in Cosmopolitan London.* New Haven & London: Yale University Press, 2012.

Finally, the research that gave rise to this book contributes to the knowledge of the British white drug subculture and its regulators. Specifically, it firstly revises the periodisation of the subculture and the surrounding regulatory architecture; secondly, it modifies our characterisation of addicts and addict subculture in the interwar decades; thirdly, it changes our understanding of the ways in which the postwar subculture arose, and its linkages and transitions with the preceding subculture. Its final contribution involves the elaboration of the chronology and dimensions of the regulatory architecture, particularly with respect to the Home Office Drugs Branch and the role of the Regional Medical Officers, and to a lesser extent the Metropolitan Police.

Bibliography

Archival Sources

TNA: The National Archives, Kew, Surrey

CRIM 1/1908, Defendant: COOPER, Wilfred and others Charge: Conspiracy to contravene the provisions of Regulation 2(1) of the Dangerous Drugs Act 1937, and unlawfully procuring drugs. Session: 1948 Mar 16.

FO 371/22204 Reports on drug addiction for League of Nations, 1938.

FO 371/23584 Reports on drug addiction for the League of Nations, 1939.

FO 371/24748 Head of Home Office Drugs Branch: appointment of Mr. Thornton, 1940.

FO 371/34548 Drug addiction in the United Kingdom in 1942, 1943.

FO 371/39379 Drug addiction in the United Kingdom in 1943, 1944.

HO 45/11285, DANGEROUS DRUGS AND POISONS: Doctors' offences, 1922–1923.

HO 45/13708, Dangerous Drugs and Poisons: Some implications of proposed Channel Tunnel (1920–1930). 'Clynes to Prime Minister, 2 June 1930'.

HO 45/18469 DANGEROUS DRUGS AND POISONS: Inspections of retail chemists: notes for the guidance of police officers, 1929–1940.

HO 45/19807 Home Office: Registered Papers. Registered Papers, 1920 onwards. DANGEROUS DRUGS AND POISONS: Dangerous Drugs (Hospital General Exemption) (Amendment) Order, 1939, 1939–1945.

C. Hallam, *White Drug Cultures and Regulation in London, 1916–1960*, https://doi.org/10.1007/978-3-319-94770-9

HO 45/19983 DANGEROUS DRUGS AND POISONS: Dangerous Drugs Acts 1920 and 1923: application to doctors and dentists; inspection of records and stocks, 1921–1929.

HO 45/20370 DANGEROUS DRUGS: General papers on application of Acts and Regulations, 1916–1946.

HO 45/20637 DANGEROUS DRUGS: Pethidine, 1942–1946.

HO 45/21172 DANGEROUS DRUGS AND POISONS: Relaxation of regulations to allow administration of morphine by approved persons in war emergency conditions. Control and storage of drugs at wartime first aid posts and in factories under government administration, 1938–1947.

HO 45/21934 DANGEROUS DRUGS: R.A.F. first-aid kits containing dangerous drugs: investigation into sale to the public, 1947–1948.

HO 45/23161 DANGEROUS DRUGS AND POISONS: Reports of losses and thefts of dangerous drugs and poisons: broadcast messages. Exclusion of dangerous drugs from RAF first-aid kits, 1946–1949.

HO 45/24761 HOME OFFICE – STAFF AND OFFICE MATTERS: Pre-war organisation of departmental drugs branch including transfer of obscene publications function, 1921–1931.

HO 45/24948, DANGEROUS DRUGS AND POISONS: Departmental Drugs Branch: annual reports, 1930–1952.

HO 45/25377 DANGEROUS DRUGS AND POISONS: Administration of morphine to air-raid casualties by rescue workers: General Medical Council and departmental memoranda, 1939–45.

HO 45/25443 DANGEROUS DRUGS AND POISONS: Dangerous Drugs Acts 1929 and 1936: contraventions by doctors; establishment of suitable tribunal, 1926–1952.

HO 144/11913 DANGEROUS DRUGS AND POISONS: Narcotic drug addiction, 1921–1930.

HO 144/11969 Dangerous Drugs and Poisons: Interpretation of Regulation 4 of Dangerous Drugs Regulations, 1921: the case stated against Dr George Chadwick Kingsbury, 1924–1930.

HO 144/20168 Dangerous Drugs and Poisons: Medical practitioners convicted under Dangerous Drugs Acts: information for use of General Medical Council, 1935–1936.

HO 144/22433 DANGEROUS DRUGS AND POISONS: Trafficking: first case of joint police action with other countries effecting simultaneous arrests in London, Montreal and Antwerp, 1932–1943.

HO 319/1 Inter-departmental Committee on Drug Addiction (Brain Committee): minutes of 1st, 2nd, 3rd and 4th meetings 1959; minutes of 1st and 2nd meetings 1960; matters arising from meetings; submission of report to Home Secretary, 1955–1961.

HO 319/2 Inter-departmental Committee on Drug Addiction (Brain Committee): Home Office evidence; addiction amongst prisoners; minutes of 2nd, 3rd and 4th meetings 1964; draft report of Committee; second report of Committee; legislation to implement recommendations, 1964–1967.
HO 319/5 Dangerous Drugs Branch: co-operation with Metropolitan Police Dangerous Drugs Squad, 1959–1966.
HO 319/14 Addiction: review of Home Office policy on drug addiction amongst authorised persons, 1953–1954.
LO 2/266 Dangerous Drugs Act 1951 S.18(1)(a): Hirschmann, J J: attorney-general: consent, 1954.
MEPO 2/4487 Illegal sales of liquor at West End night bar: imprisonment for defendant already serving sentence for drug offences, 1937.
MEPO 2/9631 Dangerous Drugs: Trafficking, Prosecution, Inspection, Lectures, 1954–1955.
MEPO 2/10167 Meetings at Home Office on the increasing use of dangerous drugs, 1962–1972.
MEPO 3/1054 Supplies of large quantities of morphine by Dr. M.D. Ripka to Brian Dean Paul, drug addict, and brother of Brenda Dean Paul, 1936–1947.
MEPO 3/1038 League of Nations Advisory Committee on traffic in opium and other dangerous drugs: quarterly summaries from July 1934–1939, 1935–1939.
MEPO 3/1093 Ms. Mock was suspected of entering into a marriage of convenience with an older man who worked as a host in a West End dance hall and was 'Associated with prostitutes and suspected drug traffickers', 1938–1939.
MEPO 3/2579 Brenda Dean Paul, Drug Addict: activities and associates 1931–1963.
MEPO 3/1023 Doctor Samuel Graham Connor: systematic treatment of a number of women for the purpose of procuring abortions (sixteen counts), 1937–1942.
MEPO 3/1056 G.E. O'Brien: sentenced to six months for possessing dangerous drugs at Lewes: particulars of conviction supplied to Institute of Chartered Accountants at their request, 1937.
MEPO 3/1673 Elvira Dolores Barney acquitted of the murder of Thomas William Scott Stephen at Williams Mews on 31 May 1932, 1932–1933.
MEPO 3/2954 Illicit trading in narcotics, 1948–1957.
MH 58/51 Dangerous Drugs Act, 1920; Regulations 1921–1926; Ministry of Health and Home Office co-operation, 1919–1927.
MH 58/565 Inter-departmental Committee on Drug Addiction: joint evidence by Home Office, Ministry of Health and Department of Health for Scotland, 1958–1960.
MH 58/270 Dangerous Drugs Act, doctors' and dentists' duties (Home Office memorandum), 1929–1938.

MH 58/277 Medical Committee on drug addiction: Evidence, 1924–1925.
MH 71/108 Committee on Drug Addiction: meetings 1–24, 1924 Nov.
MH 71/109 Committee on Drug Addiction: meetings 25–54, 1924 Dec–1925 Feb.
MH 71/110 Committee on Drug Addiction: meetings 55–90, 1925 Mar–June.
MH 76/83 'Equipment; storage of dangerous drugs', 1939–1945.
MH 135/157 Dangerous drugs: withdrawal of authority to prescribe, 1923–1957.
MH 149/166 Interdepartmental Committee on Drug Addiction: working papers, 1964–1965.

The Royal College of Physicians

11 St Andrews Place, Regents Park, LONDON NW1 4LE.
MS5911 Royal College of Physicians: *Minutes of the Committee on Drug Addiction, 1938.*

London Metropolitan Archives

LMA, 40 Northampton Road, LONDON EC1R 0HB.
A/KE/724/100/ Spelthorne St Mary, Thorpe, nr. Egham, Surrey; Community of St Mary the Virgin, Wantage; independent home for women drug and alcohol addicts and nerve cases 1955–1961.

British Library

96 Euston Road, LONDON NW1 2DB.

Wellcome Library

183 Euston Road, LONDON NW1 2BE.

Digital Archives

Ancestry UK http://www.ancestry.co.uk/
British Newspaper Archive http://www.britishnewspaperarchive.co.uk/
The Gazette: Official Public Record https://www.thegazette.co.uk/
Google Newspaper Archive https://news.google.com/newspapers
Historic Hansard 1803–2005 http://hansard.millbanksystems.com/commons/
Internet Archive https://archive.org/details/texts

Newspaper SG (Singapore and Malaya) http://eresources.nlb.gov.sg/newspapers/default.aspx
Trove Digitised Newspapers (Australia) http://trove.nla.gov.au/newspaper/
UK Press Online http://www.ukpressonline.co.uk/

Primary Sources

Government Reports and Papers

Report of the Committee Appointed by the Secretary of State for the Home Department to Consider Outstanding Objections to the Draft Regulations Under the Dangerous Drugs Act, 1920 (London: HMSO, 1921).
Departmental Committee on Morphine and Heroin Addiction: *Report* (London: HMSO, 1926).
Interdepartmental Committee on Drug Addiction: *Drug Addiction: Report of the Interdepartmental Committee* (London: HMSO, 1961).
Interdepartmental Committee on Drug Addiction: *Drug Addiction in the United Kingdom: Second Report of the Interdepartmental Committee on Drug Addiction* (London: HMSO, 1965).
Reports of the Commissioner of the Metropolitan Police, (London: HMSO, 1916 to 1966).
Report of the Royal Commission on the Law relating to Mental Illness and Mental Deficiency (London: HMSO, 1957).

Memoirs, Diaries etc.

Agnew, D. *Undercover Agent- Narcotics*. London: Souvenir Press, 1959.
Ashley, A. with Thompson, D. *The First Lady*. London: John Blake, 2006.
Baker, C. *As Though I Had Wings: The Lost Memoir*. London: Indigo, 1997.
Balfour, P. *Society Racket: A critical survey of modern social life*. London: Long, 1933.
Benney, M. *Low Company: Describing the evolution of a burglar*. Horsham: Caliban, 1981. (First published 1936).
Bestic, A. *Turn Me On Man*. London: Anthony Gibbs, Library 33, 1966.
Burke, T. *London in My Time*. Oxford: Oxford City Press, 2010. (First published 1934).
Carew, D. *The House is Gone: A Personal Retrospect*. London: Robert Hale, 1949.
Carew, D. *A Fragment of Friendship: Evelyn Waugh as a young man*. London: Everest Books, 1974.
Carlish, R. with Bestic, A. *King of Clubs*. London: Elek Books, 1962.

Carpenter, H. *The Brideshead Generation: Evelyn Waugh and His Generation.* London: Faber and Faber, 1990.
Cocteau, J. *Opium: The Diary of His Cure.* London & Chester Springs: Peter Owen, 1990. (First published 1930).
Cocteau, J. *Les Enfants Terribles.* London: Vintage, 2011. (First published 1929).
Cooper, D. *The Rainbow Comes and Goes.* London: Penguin, 1961. (First published 1958).
Daley, H. *This Small Cloud: A Personal Memoir.* London: Weidenfeld & Nicolson, 1986.
Ellis, B. & Revie, A. *I Came Back From Hell: The story of Barry Ellis.* London: Brown, Watson, 1963.
Fabian, R. *London After Dark: An intimate record of night life in London, and a selection of crime stories from the casebook of Ex-Superintendent Robert Fabian.* Kingswood, Surrey: Naldrett, 1954.
Fielding, D. *The Duchess of Jermyn Street: The Life and Good Times of Rosa Lewis of the Cavendish Hotel.* London: Eyre and Spottiswoode, 1964.
Fielding, D. Mercury Presides. London: Eyre and Spottiswoode, 1954.
Fordham, J. *Let's Join Hands and Contact the Living: Ronnie Scott and His Club.* London: Elm Tree Books, 1986.
Green, M. *Children of the Sun: A Narrative of English Decadence After 1918.* London: Pimlico, 1992. (First Published 1976).
Hahn, E. 'The Big Smoke' in O'Reilly, S. & O'Reilly, J. and Habegger, L. *Traveller's Tales: China.* San Francisco: Travellers' Tales Inc., 2000. ('The Big Smoke' first published in 1937).
Hollis, C. *Oxford in the Twenties: Recollections of five friends* London: Heinemann, 1976.
International Opium Convention of 1912 (The 'Hague Convention'), Article 9. *The American Journal of International Law*, 6 (3) Supplement: Official Documents, (1912), 177–192.
Jackson, S. *An Indiscreet Guide to Soho* London: Muse Arts Limited, 1946.
Jones, J.A. *Wonderful London Today.* London: John Long, 1934.
Kavanagh, J. *Secret Muses: The Life of Frederick Ashton.* London: Faber and Faber,1996.
King, V. *The Weeping and the Laughter: An Autobiography.* London: Macdonald and Jane's, 1976.
Lee, J.S. *Underworld of the East: Being eighteen years' actual experiences of the underworlds, drug haunts and jungles of India, China and the Malay archipelago.* London: Green Magic, 2000. (First published in 1935).
Lock, J. *Lady Policeman.* London: Michael Joseph, 1968.
Lock, J. *The British Policewoman: Her Story.* London: Robert Hale, 1979.
Mannin, E. *Julie: The Story of a Dance Hostess.* London: Hutchinson, 1940.

Mannin, E. *Young in the Twenties: A chapter of an autobiography.* London: Hutchinson, 1971.

Major, J.W. *Quayside Crooks.* London: Stanley Paul, 1941.

Meyrick, K. *Secrets of the 43 Club.* Dublin: Parkgate, 1994. (First published 1933).

Mezzrow, M. & Wolfe, B. *Really the Blues.* New York: Random House, 1946.

Morain, A. *The Underworld of Paris: Secrets of the Sureté.* New York: Blue Ribbon Books, 1931.

Paul, B.D. *My First Life: A biography.* London: Dent, 1935.

Sergre, D. writing as 'Pitigrilli' *Cocaine.* Feltham: Hamlyn Paperbacks, 1982. (First published in 1921).

Thorpe, R. *Viper: The Confessions of a Drug Addict.* London: Robert Hale, 1956.

Tietjen, A. *Soho: London's Vicious Circle.* London: Allen Wingate, 1956.

Viator, 'When the D. D. A. Licence is Withdrawn' Chemist *and Druggist* 122, 2883 (1935) 572.

Waugh, A. *A Year to Remember: a reminiscence of 1931.* London: W. H. Allen, 1975.

Wishart, M. *High Diver: An Autobiography.* London: Quartet Books, 1978.

Wyles, L. *A Woman at Scotland Yard.* London: Faber and Faber, 1952.

Wyndham, F. *Mrs Henderson.* New York: Moyer Bell, 1985.

Contemporary Journals

Anon. 'Case under the Dangerous Drugs Regulations' *British Medical Journal*: Supplement 1144 (1926a) 213–215.

Anon. 'Dangerous Drugs Acts' *Chemist & Druggist* 118,2765 (1933) 108.

Anon. 'Disciplinary Cases' *British Medical Journal* 2,2971, (1917) 113–115.

Anon. 'Drug Addiction', *The Lancet* 233,6038 (1939) 1156–1157.

Anon. 'Failure to Comply with Dangerous Drugs Regulations' *British Medical Journal* 2,3588 (1929), 694.

Anon. 'Medicine and the Law: Prison or Hospital for Drug Addict?' *Lancet* 232,5999 (1938) 454–455.

Anon. 'Medical Notes in Parliament', *British Medical Journal* 2,3993 (1937) 144–146.

Anon. 'Medico-Legal' *British Medical Journal* 1,3406, (1926b), 677–678.

Anon, 'Medico-Legal: Drug Summons Dismissed' *British Medical Journal* 2,4942 (1955) 797.

Anon. 'Medico-Legal Society' *Lancet* 217, 5623 (1931) 1241–1243.

Anon. 'Penal Cases: Case of Samuel Grahame Connor' *The Lancet* 207,5363 (1926), 1147–1150.

Anon. 'Prevention and Treatment of Drug Addiction', *The Lancet* 217,5611 (1931) 587–588.

Anon. The International Opium Convention, article IX, in The *American Journal of International Law*, 6,3, Supplement: Official Documents, (1912) 177–192.

Anon. 'Offences in respect of Dangerous Drugs' *British Medical Journal*, 2,3961, Supplement, 5 December (1936) 310.

A member of the community of St Mary the Virgin, 'The Moral, Mental and Physical Background of Female Inebriates', *British Journal of Inebriety* 42,1 (1944) 3–20.

Adams, E.W. 'Some Unusual Forms of Drug Addiction', *British Journal of Inebriety*, 31,1, (1933) 1–15.

Adams, E.W. 'What Is Addiction?' *British Journal of Inebriety*, 34,1 (1935) 1–11.

Cooke, E. 'The Drug Squad' *Journal of Forensic Science* 3, (1962) 43–48.

Delevingne, M. 'Some international aspects of the problem of drug addiction' *British Journal of Addiction,* 32,3 (1935) 125–151.

Dixon, W.E. 'A Clinical Address On Drug Addiction. Given At The Annual Meeting Of The British Medical Association, Winnipeg, August, 1930', *British Medical Journal*, 2,3634, (1930) 19–24.

Frankau, I.M. & Stanwell, P.M. 'Treatment of Drug-Addiction' *The Lancet,* 276, 7165 (1960) 1377–1379.

Frankau, I.M. & Stanwell, P.M. 'Treatment of Drug Addiction' (letter) *The Lancet*, 277,7171 (1961) 279–280.

Hamill, P. 'Morphine Injection at First Aid Posts' Lancet 233,6038 (1939) 1139–1192.

Frankau, Lady. 'Treatment in England of Canadian Patients Addicted to Narcotic Drugs' *Canadian Medical Association Journal*, 90, (1964) 421–424.

Lyle, G. 'Dangerous Drug Traffic in London' *British Journal of Addiction* 50,1 (1953) 47–55.

Norwood East, W. 'The Problem of Alcohol and Drug Addiction in Relation to Crime', *British Journal of Inebriety* 37,2 (1939) 55–73.

Reid, J. 'The Treatment of Female Inebriates and Drug Addicts' *British Journal of Inebriety* 24,2 (1926) 58–62.

Rootham, H. 'Jazzomania and Devil Dances' *English Review* (January 1924) 109–111.

Sharkey, S. 'Morphinomania' *Nineteenth Century: a monthly review*, 127 (1887) 335–342.

Tudor- Hart, J. 'Drug Addiction' (letter) *British Medical Journal*, 270,6992 (1957), 468.

Viator, 'When the D. D. A. Licence is Withdrawn' Chemist *and Druggist* 122,2883 (1935) 572.

Waddington, I. 'The professionalisation of medicine', *British Medical Journal* 301, 6754 (1990), 688–690.

Whippell Gadd, H. 'The ownership of medical prescriptions', *The Lancet* 176, 4544 (1910), 1030.

Willcox, W. 'Norman Kerr Memorial Lecture on Drug Addiction', *British Medical Journal* 2,3283 (1923) 1013–1018.
Willcox, W. 'Medico-legal aspects of alcohol and drug addiction' *British Journal of Inebriety* 31,4 (1934) 131–144.
Wolff, P. 'Alcohol and Drug Addiction in Germany: Part 2- Drug Addiction' *British Journal of Inebriety* 30, (4) (1933) 160–171

Contemporary Newspapers

Times, Daily Mail, Daily Express, Daily Mirror, News of the World, Guardian, Daily Telegraph, Sunday Dispatch, Morning Advertiser, Yorkshire Post, Yorkshire Evening Post, Glasgow Herald, Western Daily Press, Gloucester Citizen, Gloucestershire Echo, Daily Record, Birmingham Daily Post, Aberdeen Press & Journal, Dundee Evening Telegraph
'12 on Drug Charges' *The Gloucester Citizen* 15 April 1950, 1.
'£200 Fine and Six Months for London Doctor' *Dundee Evening Telegraph,* 29 March 1926, 7.
'£7,000 A-Year Man Acquitted' *Hull Daily Mail* 26 March 1935,12.
'£10,000 A Year Man Ran Nightclubs' *Daily Express* 8 July 1937, 9.
'A Story of Drug-taking' *Birmingham Daily Post* 16 July 1917, 7.
'A Woman P.C.'s Drinks' *Daily Mirror* 15 August 1932, 4.
'Babette's Last Letter Before Death Leap' *Daily Mail* 31 August 1932, 5.
'Borstal for Playboy Forger' *Daily Mirror*, 10 March 1938, 9.
'"Bottle Party" Case' *Times* 17 September 1932, 17.
'Bottle Party System Legal' *Gloucester Citizen* 28 July 1933, 10.
'Bought Heroin, Court Told' Daily *Mirror*, 21 February 1947, 3.
'Brenda Dean Paul in Drug Case' *Daily Mirror* 23 August 1932, 5.
'Brenda Paul Fit to be Liberated: Famous Doctors to be Called in Drug Case' *Daily Express* 9 March 1933, 3.
'Brilliant young man in West End toils', *News of the World*, 11 July 1937, 5.
'Business Offers' *Times* 17 March 1933, 1.
'Club Struck Off the Register' *Times* 20th April 1932, 11.
'Conviction for Drugs Offence' *Times* 16 March 1938, 9.
'Cured of Drug Addiction' *Times* 18 October 1937, 11.
'Dance Hostess System Attacked by Judge' *Daily Mirror* 20 November 1931, 2.
'Dancer as "Slave of Hashish"' *Daily Mail* 11 October 1937, 8.
'Dancing, Dope and Death' *Daily Express* 11 March 1922, 1.
'Dangerous Drug in Woman's Flat' *Times* 13 October 1938, 4.
'Dangerous Drugs Prosecution' *Times* 7 December 1931, 7.
'Dangerous Drugs Regulations' *Times* 2 March 1926, 6.
'Doctor Cleared in Drug Case' *Daily Mirror* 9 September 1955, 5.

'Doctor fined £300 for Helping Woman to get Drugs' *Daily Express* 12 February 1953, 5.
'Doctor's Name Removed from the Register' *Birmingham Daily Post* 30 November 1917, 7.
'Dope: A personal story is today's documentary evidence in a nation-wide Daily Express Drug Investigation' *Daily Express* 28 November 1951, 3.
'Dope Trade Revelation' *Daily Express* 15 May 1930, 11.
'Dope –Vilest of All the Rackets' *Daily Mirror* 26 March 1947, 2.
'Driven Mad by Hashish' *Daily Express* 6 November 1930, 8.
'Dr. Starkie Sent to Prison' *Times* 17 September 1921, 5.
'Drug Addict's Doctor Fined' *Daily Telegraph* 12 February 1953, 9.
'Drug Addict's Suicide' *Times* 31 August 1932, 7.
'Drugs in West-End Flat' *Times* 2 June 1923,9.
'Drugs in Woman's Flat' *Times 11 October 1937, 9.*
'Drug Summons Dismissed' *Times* 9 September 1955, 5.
'Drug Taker is "Through with Night Club Life"' *Daily Express* 18 October 1937, 5.
'Drug Treatment: Doctor's Explanation in Court' *Yorkshire Post* 31 January 1933, 5.
'Drugs Were "Planted" on Music Hall Star' *Daily Mail* 16 March 1938, 9.
'Ex-Doctor Sent to Prison' *Times* 3 December 1929, 11.
'Friends Made Her a Drug Addict' *Daily Express* 13 October 1938,13.
'Gaol for Doctor' *Daily Mirror* 30 March 1926, 18.
'Gaol Sentence on Doctor' *Daily Mail* 30 March 1926, 8.
'Girl's Ruse to Get Drugs' *Daily Mirror* 7 December 1931, 6.
'Girl Victim of Drugs' *Daily Express* 7 December 1931, 7.
'Girl Victim of "Pernicious Beast"' *News of the World* 10 October 1937, 2.
'Haunts of the "Reefer"' *Times*, 15 July 1957, 11.
'High Court of Justice: Kings Bench Division: Kingsbury vs, Director of Public Prosecutions' *Times* 11 November 1926, 5.
'Hospital had a Special "Raid Warning"' *Daily Mirror*, 7 September 1943, 1.
'Hostess of a "Bottle Party"' *Daily Mirror* 17 September 1932, 5.
'Illegal Supplying of Morphine' *Times* 30 March 1926,11.
'Illegal Supplying of Morphine' *Times* 17 April 1926, 9.
'I've Finished With Dope' *Daily Mail* 18 October 1937, 9.
'Jewel Robbery Charge' *Times*, 16 February 1938, 18.
'Liquor at "Bottle Parties"' *Times* 15 August 1932, 7.
'Liquor Sales at West End Night Bar Were Illegal' *Morning Advertiser*, 23 October 1937, n.p.
'Mayfair Playboys, Too Poor for Luxury Lives, Took to Crime' *Daily Mirror* 19 February 1938, 3, *passim.*
'Medicine Cure For Crime' *Gloucestershire Echo* 25 November 1933, 1.

'Menace of Bottle Parties' *Perth Sunday Times* 23 January 1938, 5.
'Mental Hygiene: National Council Formed' *Times*, 5 May 1922, 18.
'Miss Brenda Dean Paul Charged' *Times* 23 August 1932, 7.
'Miss Cissie Loftus Charged' *Times* 11 November 1922, 7.
'Money Raised on Jewellery' *Times* 13 March 1935, 8.
'Morphine Victims' *Times* 27 August 1924, 7.
'Mrs. A. R. Carew Sent to a Nursing Home' *Daily Express* 10 September 1932, 7.
'New Life for Brenda Dean Paul' *Daily Mirror* 12 November 1932, 16.
'Opium Traffic: Man and Woman Sentenced' *Times* 8 January 1923, 7.
'Playboy Gangsters Had Flight Planned' *Daily Express* 19 February 1938, 1, *passim*.
'Police Raid on Hotel' *Times*, 7 December 1936, 11.
'Policeman's Champagne at a "Bottle Party"' *Daily Mirror* 6 August 1932, 7.
'Possession of Drugs' *Times* 28 May 1923, 7.
'"Prince" Drug Pedlar Guilty' *Daily Mail* 12 July 1949, 7.
'Promotions at Scotland Yard' *Times* 2 August 1929, 14.
'Saturated with Drugs' *Aberdeen Press and Journal*, 2 June 1923, 8.
'Smuggling of Drugs' Times 28 June 1932, 11.
'State Homes for Drug Victims' *Daily Express* 13 March 1931, 7.
'Street Offences' *Times* 3 December 1927, 4.
'Talk of London' *Daily Express* 6 August 1932, 13.
'The Face of a Dope-Party Girl' *Daily Express* 07 March 1952, 3.
'The Man Who "Put His Soul in Pawn"' *Daily Express* 18 October 1951, 5.
'The tragedy that was Brenda Dean Paul' *Daily Express* 27 July 1959, 1.
'"These will make your mouth water"– drug charge story' *Daily Mirror* 5 May 1949, 1.
'Victim of a Beast' *Daily Express* 14 October 1937, 1.
'William Hickey column' *Daily Express* 9 September 1938, 6.
'Woman on Bilking Charge' *Times* 1 November 1939, 3.
'Youths Struggle to See Miss Dean Paul' *Western Daily Press* 6 September 1932, 5.

Secondary Sources

Books and Journals

Acker, C. *Creating the American Junkie: Addiction Research in the Classic Era of Narcotic Control.* Baltimore: The Johns Hopkins University Press, 2002.
Addison, P. *No Turning Back: The Peacetime Revolutions of Post-War Britain* Oxford: Oxford University Press, 2010.

Alexander, S. 'A New Civilization? London Surveyed 1928–1940s' *History Workshop Journal*, 64, (2007).

Anderson, S. & Berridge, V. 'Opium in 20th century Britain: pharmacists, regulation and the people' Addiction, 95,1 (2000) 23–36.

Anon. 'Providing the capital with a 24-hour service', *Chemist & Druggist*, 202,4941 (1974) 768–769.

Anon. 'Scots Cop founded the UK's first drug unit: How George Lyle fought menace' *Daily Record*, 31 July (2012).

Armstrong, D. *The Political anatomy of the body: medical knowledge in Britain in the twentieth century.* Cambridge: Cambridge University Press, 1983.

Barrow, A. *Gossip: A History of High Society from 1920 to 1970.* London: Hamish Hamilton, 1978.

Bean, P. *The Social Control of Drugs.* London: Wiley Blackwell, 1968.

Bean, P. (ed.) *Cocaine and Crack: Supply and Use.* New York: St Martin's Press, 1993.

Bean, P. 'Policing the Medical Profession: The Use of Tribunals' in Whynes, D.K. & Bean, P. (eds.) *Policing and Prescribing: The British System of Drug Control.* Basingstoke, Hampshire: Macmillan, 1991.

Becker, H. *Outsiders: Studies in the Sociology of Deviance.* New York: Simon & Schuster, 1997. (First published 1963).

Bennett, A. & Harris, K. (eds.) *After Subculture: Critical Studies in Contemporary Youth Culture Andy Bennett and Keith Harris.* London: Palgrave/Macmillan, 2004.

Benson, J. *The Rise of Consumer Society in Britain 1880–1980.* London: Longman, 1994.

Berridge, V. 'War conditions and narcotics control: the passing of the Defence of the Realm Act regulation 40B' *Journal of Social Policy*, 7, (1978) 285–304.

Berridge, V. 'East End opium dens and narcotic use in Britain' London *Journal* 4,1 (1978) 3–28.

Berridge, V. 'Professionalization and narcotics: the medical and pharmaceutical professions and British narcotic use 1868–1926' *Psychological Medicine* 8,3 (1978) 361–372.

Berridge, V. 'Drugs and Social Policy: The Establishment of Drug Control in Britain 1900–1930' *British Journal of Addiction*, 79 (1984) 17–29.

Berridge, V. 'The Origins of the English Drug "Scene" 1890–1930' *Medical History*, 32 (1988) 51–64.

Berridge, V. 'The Society for the Study of Addiction 1884–1988' Supplement to *British Journal of Addiction*, 85,8 (1990).

Berridge, V. 'Doctors and the State: The Changing Role of Medical Expertise in Policy-Making' *Contemporary British History*, 11,4 (1997) 66–85.

Berridge, V. "'Stamping out addiction': the work of the Rolleston Committee 1924–1926' in Berrios, G.E. & Freeman, H. (eds.) *150 Years of British Psychiatry Volume 2: The Aftermath*. London: Athlone, 1996.

Berridge, V. *Opium and the People: Opiate Use and Drug Control Policy in Nineteenth and Early Twentieth Century England*. London: Free Association Books, 1999.

Berridge, V. 'Punishment or Treatment? Inebriety, Drink, and Drugs 1860–2004', The *Lancet* 364, Supplement 1 (2004).

Berridge, V. 'The British System and its History: Myth and Reality' in Strang, J. & Gossop, M. (eds.) *Heroin Addiction and the British System: Volume 1: Origins and Evolution*. Abingdon: Routledge, 2005. 7–16.

Berridge, V. 'Heroin Prescription and History' *New England Journal of Medicine* 361,8 (2009) 280–821.

Berridge, V. *Demons: Our changing attitudes to alcohol, tobacco and drugs*. Oxford: Oxford University Press, 2013.

Bewley, T. 'Recent changes in the pattern of drug abuse in the United Kingdom' *Bulletin on narcotics*, 4, (1966) 1–14.

Bewley, T. 'The drugs problem of the 1960s: A new type of problem' in Strang, J. & Gossop, M. (eds.) *Heroin Addiction and the British System: Origins and Evolution*. Abingdon: Routledge, 2005. 43–52.

Bewley-Taylor, D.R. *The United States and International Drug Control, 1909–1997*. London: Continuum, 2001.

Bingham, A. *Gender, Modernity and the Popular Press in Interwar Britain*. Oxford: Oxford University Press, 2004.

Bingham, A. *Family Newspapers: Sex, Private Life, and the British Popular Press 1918–1978*. Oxford: Oxford University Press, 2009.

Bishop, 'Willcox, Sir William Henry (1870–1941)', rev. K.D. Watson, *Oxford Dictionary of National Biography*, Oxford: Oxford University Press, 2004.

Blackman, S. 'Youth Subculture Theory: A Critical Engagement with the Concept, its Origins and Politics, from the Chicago School to Postmodernism' *Journal of Youth Studies*, 8,1 (2005) 1–20.

Blackwell, J. 'The Saboteurs of Britain's Opiate Policy: Overprescribing Physicians or American-Style 'Junkies'?' *The International Journal of the Addictions*, 23,5 (1988) 517–526.

Blake, A. 'Mental health and moral panic: drug discourses in history' in Manning, P. (ed.) *Drugs and Popular Culture: Drugs, media and identity in contemporary society*. Devon: Willan Publishing, 2007.

Bland, L. '"Guardians of the Race" or "Vampires on the Nation's Health"?' in Whitelegg, E., Arnot, M., Bartels, E., Beechey, V., Birke, L., Himmelweit, S., Leonard, D., Ruehl, S. & Speakman, M.A. (eds.) *The Changing Experience of Women*. Oxford: Martin Robinson, 1982.

Bland, L. 'White Women and Men of Colour: Miscegenation Fears in Britain after the Great War' *Gender and History,* 17,1 (2005) 29–61.

Bland, L. *Modern Women on Trial: Sexual Transgression in the Age of the Flapper.* Manchester: Manchester University Press, 2013.

Block, A. 'European Drug Trafficking and Traffickers between the Wars: The Policy of Suppression and its Consequences' *Journal of Social History,* 23,2 (1989) 315–337.

Blondel, N. *The Journals of Mary Butts: Henry McBride Series in Modernism and Modernity.* New Haven: Yale University Press, 2003.

Blue, G. 'Opium for China: The British Connection' in Brook, T. & Wakabayashi, B.T. *Opium Regimes: China, Britain and Japan, 1839–1952.* London: University of California Press, 2000.

Blythe, R. *The Age of Illusion: England in the Twenties and Thirties 1919–40.* Harmondsworth: Penguin, 1963.

Booth, M. *A Magick Life: A Biography of Aleister Crowley* London: Stodder and Houghton, 2001.

Bosanquet, N. & Salisbury, C. 'The Practice' in Loudon, I., Horder, J. & Webster, C. *General Practice under the National Health Service, 1948–1997.* London: Clarendon Press, 1998.

Breward, C. *Fashion.* Oxford: Oxford University Press, 2003.

Breese, C. *Hutch.* London: Bloomsbury, 1999.

Bridge, W. *Captain Henry Evelyn Arthur Platt – Diaries and Letters of a First World War Officer.* CreateSpace Independent Publishing Platform, 2012.

Brivati, B. & Jones, H. (eds.) *What Difference Did The War Make?* London: Leicester University Press, 1993.

Brook, T. & Wakabayashi, T. (eds.) *Opium Regimes: China, Britain and Japan, 1839–1952.* Berkeley, Los Angeles and London: University of California, 2000.

Brooker, P. *Bohemia in London: The Social Scene of Early Modernism.* Basingstoke: Palgrave Macmillan, 2007.

Browne, D.G. *Bernard Spilsbury: His Life and Cases.* London: George G. Harrap, 1951.

Bruun, K., Pan, L. & Rexed, I. *The Gentlemen's Club: International Control of Drugs and Alcohol.* Chicago: University of Chicago, 1975.

Buxton, J. *The Political Economy of Narcotics: Production, Consumption & Global Markets.* London and New York: Zedbooks, 2006.

Campbell, A. & Niel, T. *A Life In Pieces: Reflections on Alexander Trocchi.* Edinburgh: Rebel Inc., 1997.

Campbell, C. *The Romantic Ethic and the Spirit of Modern Consumerism.* Alcuin Academics, 2005. (First published in 1987).

Cannadine, D. *The Decline and Fall of the British Aristocracy.* London: Papermac, 1996.

Chandler, D. *Semiotics: The Basics.* London: Routledge, 2007.

Chouvy, P.A. *Opium: Uncovering the Politics of the Poppy.* London: I.B. Tauris, 2009.

Conekin, B., Mort, F. & Waters, C. (eds.) *Moments of Modernity: Reconstructing Britain 1945–1964.* London & New York: Rivers Oram Press, 1999.

Cotes, P. *Trial of Elvira Barney* London: David & Charles, 1976.

Courtwright, F.D. 'The Roads to H: The Emergence of the American Heroin Complex, 1898–1956' in Musto D.F. (ed.) *One Hundred Years of Heroin.* Westport, Connecticut; London: Auburn House, 2002.

Courtwright, D.T. *Forces of Habit: Drugs and the Making of the Modern World.* Cambridge: Harvard University Press, 2001.

Davenport-Hines, R. *The Pursuit of Oblivion: A Global History of Narcotics 1500–2000.* London: Weidenfeld & Nicolson, 2001.

Davenport-Hines, R. *An English Affair: Sex, Class and Power in the Age of Profumo.* London: Harper Press, 2013.

Davie, M. (ed.) *The Diaries of Evelyn Waugh.* London: Phoenix, 1995.

Derrida, J. 'The Rhetoric of Drugs' in Alexander, A. & Roberts, M.S. (eds.) *High Culture: reflections on addiction and modernity.* Albany: State University of New York Press, 1989 19–42.

Digby, A. & Bosanquet, N. 'Doctors and patients in an era of national health insurance and private practice, 1913–1938' *Economic History Review* 2nd series, XLI (1988) 74–94.

Digby, A. *The Evolution of British General Practice 1850–1948.* Oxford: Oxford University Press, 1999.

Donnelly, M. *Britain in the Second World War.* London: Routledge, 1999.

Donnelly, M. *Sixties Britain: Culture, Society and Politics.* Harlow: Longman, 2005.

Downes, D. *Contrasts in Tolerance: Post War Penal Policy in the Netherlands and in England and Wales.* Oxford: Clarendon Press, 1993.

Downes, D. *The Delinquent Solution: A Study in Subcultural Theory.* Abingdon: Routledge, 2005.

Dyhouse, C. *Glamour: Women, History, Feminism.* London: Zed Books, 2010.

Dyhouse, C. *Girl Trouble: Panic and Progress in the History of Young Women.* London: Zed Books, 2013.

Emsley, C. *The English Police: A Political and Social History- Second Edition.* Edinburgh: Pearson Education, 1996.

Emsley, C. *The Great British Bobby: A History of British Policing from the 18th Century to the Present.* London: Quercus, 2009.

Emsley, C. *Crime and Society in Twentieth-Century England.* Harlow: Pearson Education, 2011.

Faulks, S. *The Fatal Englishman: Three Short Lives.* London: Vintage, 1997.

Ferris, P. *The Nameless: Abortion in Britain Today.* London: Pelican, 1967.

Fitzgerald, F. *Just Garret.* Dublin: Liberties Press, 2011.

Foucault, M. edited by Rabinow, P. *The Foucault Reader* London: Penguin, 1984.
Foucault, M. & (ed.) Gordon, C. *Power/Knowledge: Selected interviews and other writings, 1972–77.* London: Longman, 1995.
Foucault, M. *The Archaeology of Knowledge.* Routledge: London, 1989.
Foucault, M. *Discipline and Punish: The Birth of the Prison.* London: Penguin Books, 1991.
Foucault, M. *The Will to Knowledge: The History of Sexuality Volume 1.* London: Penguin Books, 1998.
Fowler, D. *The First Teenagers: The Lifestyle of Young Wage-Earners in Interwar Britain.* London: Woburn Press, 1995.
Fowler, D. *Youth Culture in Modern Britain, c. 1920–1970: From Ivory Tower to Global Movement- A New History.* Basingstoke: Palgrave Macmillan, 2008.
Fox, J. *White Mischief.* London: Vintage, 1998.
Galliher, J.F., Keys, D.P. & Elsner, E. 'Lindesmith v. Anslinger: An Early Government Victory in the Failed War on Drugs.' *The Journal of Criminal Law and Criminology*, 88, (1998) 661–682.
Gardiner, J. *Wartime: Britain 1939–1945.* London: Headline, 2004.
Gardiner, J. *The Thirties: An Intimate History of Britain.* London: Harper, 2010.
Garland, D. *Punishment and Welfare: A History of Penal Strategies.* Aldershot: Gower, 1985.
Gelder, K. (ed.) *The Subcultures Reader, Second Edition.* London: Routledge, 2005.
Gillespie, D., Glatt, M.M., Hills, D.R. & Pittman, D.J. 'Drug Dependence and Abuse in England' *British Journal of Addiction to Alcohol and Other Drugs*, 62,1–2 (1967) 155–170.
Godbolt, J. *A History of Jazz in Britain 1919–1950.* London: Northway Publications, 2010.
Graves, R. & Hodge, A. *The Long Weekend: The Living Story of the Twenties and Thirties.* Harmondsworth: Penguin, 1970. (First published in 1940).
Grayzel, S.R. *At Home and Under Fire: Air Raids and Culture in Britain from the Great War to the Blitz.* Cambridge: Cambridge University Press, 2012.
Green, M. *Children of the Sun: A Narrative of Decadence in England After 1918.* London: Constable, 1977.
Gundle, S. *Glamour: A History.* Oxford: Oxford University Press, 2008.
Hall, L.A. *Sex, Gender and Social Change in Britain since 1880.* Basingstoke & London: Macmillan Press, 2000.
Hall, S. & Jefferson, T. (eds.) *Resistance through Rituals: youth subcultures in post-war Britain (2nd edition).* London and New York: Routledge, 2006.
Hankey, J. *A Passion for Egypt: Arthur Weigall, Tutankhamun and the 'Curse of the Pharaohs'.* London: Tauris Peake Paperbacks, 2007.
Hebdige, R. *Subculture: The Meaning of Style.* London: Methuen, 1979.
Heining, D. *Trad Dads, Dirty Boppers and Free Fusioneers: British Jazz, 1960–1975.* Sheffield: Equinox Publishing, 2012.

Hewison, R. *Under Siege: Literary Life in London 1939–1945*. Newton Abbott: Readers Union, 1978.

Hoare, P. 'Paul, Brenda Irene Isabelle Frances Theresa Dean (1907–1959)', *Oxford Dictionary of National Biography*. Oxford: Oxford University Press, 2004.

Honigsbaum, F. *The division in British medicine: a history of the separation of general practice from hospital care, 1911–1968*. New York: St Martin's Press, 1979.

Horn, A. *Juke Box Britain: Americanisation and youth culture, 1945–1960*. Manchester: University Press, 2009.

Horn, P. *Flappers: The real lives of British women in the era of The Great Gatsby*. Stroud: Amberley, 2013.

Horn, P. *Country House Society: The private lives of England's upper class after the First World War*. Stroud: Amberley, 2013.

Horwood, C. *Keeping Up Appearances: Fashion and Class Between the Wars*. Stroud: The History Press, 2011.

Houlbrook, M. *Queer London: Perils and Pleasures in the Sexual Metropolis, 1918–1957*. London: University of Chicago Press, 2005.

Humphrey, C. 'Place, Space and Reputation: The Changing Role of Harley Street in English Health Care' Social *Theory and Health* 2,2 (2004) 153–169.

Jackson, L.A. "Lady Cops' and 'DecoyDoras': Gender, Surveillance and the Construction of Urban Knowledge 1919–59' *London Journal*, 27,1 (2002).

Jackson, L.A. *Women Police: Gender, Welfare and Surveillance in the Twentieth Century*. Manchester: Manchester University Press, 2006.

Jeffery, C.G. 'Drug Control in the United Kingdom' in Phillipson, R.V. (ed.) *Modern Trends in Drug Dependence and Alcoholism*. London: Butterworths, 1970. 60–89.

Jeffreys, M. 'General Practitioners and the Other Caring Professions', in Loudon, I., Horder, J. & Webster, C. (eds.) *General Practice under the National Health Service, 1948–1997*. London, Clarendon Press, 1998. 128–145.

Jenkins, A. *The Twenties*. London: Heinemann, 1974.

Jenkins, A. *The Thirties*. London: Heinemann, 1976.

Jerram, L. *Streetlife: The untold story of Europe's twentieth century*. Oxford: Oxford University Press, 2011.

Joan Elizabeth, Sister 'Helping Women Addicts at Spelthorne St Mary's, England' *International Journal of Offender Therapy and Comparative Criminology*, 18 (1974) 77–81.

Judson, H.F. *Heroin Addiction in Britain: What Americans can learn from the English experience*. London and New York: Harcourt Brace, 1974.

Kavanagh, J. *Secret Muses: The Life of Frederick Ashton*. London: Faber & Faber, 1996.

Kennedy, C. *Mayfair: A Social History*. London: Hutchinson, 1986.

Knepper, P. *International Crime in the 20th Century: The League of Nations Era, 1919–1939*. Basingstoke: Palgrave Macmillan, 2011.

Kohn, M. *Narcomania: On Heroin*. London: Faber and Faber, 1987.

Kohn, M. 'Life and Times: Grains of Truth' *The Guardian*, September 1st (1990).

Kohn, M. 'Cocaine girls: sex, drugs and modernity in London during and after the First World War' in Gootenberg, P. (ed.) *Cocaine: Global Histories*. London and New York: Routledge, 1999.

Kohn, M. *Dope Girls: The Birth of the British Drug Underground*. London: Granta Books, 2001.

Kynaston, D. *Austerity Britain 1945–51*. London: Bloomsbury, 2007.

Laite, J. *Common Prostitutes and Ordinary Citizens: Commercial Sex in London, 1885–1960*. Basingstoke: Palgrave Macmillan, 2011.

Lancaster, M.J. *Brian Howard: Portrait of a Failure*. London: Timewell Press, 2005.

Lart, R. 'Medical Power and Knowledge: The Treatment and Control of Drugs and Drug Users' in Coomber, R. (ed.) *The Control of Drugs and Drug Users: Reason or Reaction?* Amsterdam: Harwood Academic Publishers, 1998.

Lawrence, C. 'Edward Jenner's Jockey Boots and the Great Tradition in English Medicine 1918–1939' in Lawrence, C. & Mayer, A.K. (eds.) *Regenerating England: Science, Medicine and Culture in Inter-War Britain*. Amsterdam-Atlanta, GA: Editions Rodopi B.V., 2000.

Leech, K. *Keep the Faith, Baby: A close-up of London's drop-outs*. London: S.P.C.K., 1973.

Leech, K. 'The Junkies' Doctors and the London Drug Scene in the 1960s: Some Remembered Fragments' in Whynes, D.K. & Bean, P. (eds.) *Policing and Prescribing: The British System of Drug Control*. Basingstoke, Hampshire: Macmillan, 1991.

Lindesmith, A.R. 'The Argot of the Underworld Drug Addict' *Journal of Criminal Law and Criminology*, 29,2 (1938) 261–278.

Lock, J. *The British Policewoman: Her Story*. London: Robert Hale, 1978.

Lock, J. *Lady Policeman*. London: Michael Joseph, 1968.

Lock, J. *Marlborough Street: The Story of a London Court*. London: Robert Hale, 1980.

Loudon, I. *Medical Care and the General Practitioner, 1750–1850*. Oxford: Clarendon Press, 1986.

Loudon, I., Horder, J. & Webster, C. *General Practice under the National Health Service, 1948–1997*. London: Clarendon Press, 1998.

Luke, M. *David Tennant and the Gargoyle Years*. London: Weidenfeld and Nicolson, 1991.

Lycett, A. *Dylan Thomas: A New Life*. London: Phoenix, 2004.

Mackay, R. *Half the Battle: Civilian Morale in Britain During the Second World War*. Manchester: Manchester University Press, 2002.

Malcolm, M.T. 'Morphine Withdrawal, Treatments 1900–1930' History *of Psychiatry*,10,37 (1999) 13–26.

Manning, P. 'An introduction to theoretical approaches and research traditions' in Manning, Paul (ed.) *Drugs and Popular Culture: Drugs, media and identity in contemporary society.* Devon: Willan Publishing, 2007.

Mars, Sarah G. *The Politics of Addiction: Medical Conflict and Drug Dependence in England since the 1960s.* Basingstoke: Palgrave Macmillan, 2012.

McAllister, W.B. *Drug Diplomacy in the Twentieth Century: An international history.* London and New York: Routledge, 2000.

McKibbin, R. *Classes and Cultures: England 1918–1951.* Oxford: Oxford University Press, 2000.

McLaren, A. *Twentieth-Century Sexuality: A History.* Oxford: Blackwell, 1999.

McLaren, A. *Playboys & Mayfair Men: Crime, Class, Masculinity, and Fascism in 1930s London* Baltimore, Johns Hopkins Press, 2017.

McCoy, A.W. *The Politics of Heroin: CIA Complicity in the Global Drugs Trade.* Chicago: Lawrence Hill, 2003.

Melman, B. *Women and the Popular Imagination in the Twenties: Flappers and Nymphs.* New York: St Martin's Press, 1988.

Meyer, K. & Parssinen, T. *Webs of Smoke: Smugglers, Warlords, Spies, and the History of the International Drug Trade.* Oxford: Rowman and Littlefield, 1998.

Mills, J.H. *Cannabis Britannica: Empire, Trade and Prohibition.* Oxford: Oxford University Press, 2003.

Mills, J.H. *Cannabis Nation: Control and Consumption in Britain, 1928–2008.* Oxford: Oxford University Press, 2012.

Mold, A. *Heroin: The Treatment of Addiction in Twentieth-Century Britain.* Dekalb, Illinois: Northern Illinois University Press, 2008.

Mooney, D. 'Poldowski Rediscovered' *Dublin Institute of Technology* http://arrow.dit.ie/aaconmusart/4/

Mort, F. *Capital Affairs: London and the Making of the Permissive Society.* New Haven & London: Yale University Press, 2010.

Muggleton, D. *Inside Subculture: The Postmodern Meaning of Style.* Oxford: Berg, 2000.

Muggleton, D. 'From classlessness to clubculture: A genealogy of post-war British youth cultural analysis' *Young,* 13 (2005) 205–219.

Musto, D.F. *The American Disease: Origins of Narcotic Control.* New York: Oxford University Press, 1987.

Nicholson, V. *Among the Bohemians: Experiments in Living 1900–1939.* London: Penguin, 2002.

Overy, R. *The Morbid Age: Britain and the Crisis of Civilization, 1919–1939.* Penguin: London, 2009.

Padwa, H. *Social Poison: The Culture and Politics of Opiate Control in Britain and France, 1891–1926.* Baltimore: Johns Hopkins University Press, 2012.

Parsonage, C. *The Evolution of Jazz in Britain, 1880–1935.* Aldershot: Ashgate, 2005.

Parssinen, T.M. *Secret Passions, Secret Remedies: Narcotic drugs in British Society 1820–1930*. Philadelphia: Institute for the Study of Human Issues, 1983.

Perkin, Harold. *The Rise of Professional Society: England since 1880*. Abingdon: Routledge, 1989.

Petrow, S. *Policing Morals: the Metropolitan Police and the Home Office, 1870–1914*. Oxford: Clarendon Press, 1994.

Plant, S. *Writing on Drugs*. London: Faber and Faber, 1999.

Playfair, G. *Six Studies in Hypocrisy*. London: Secker & Warburg, 1969.

Porter, D. 'Eugenics and the Sterilisation Debate in Sweden and Britain before World War Two' *Scandinavian Journal of History* 24,2 (1999) 145-162.

Pugh, M. *'We Danced All Night': A Social History of Britain Between the Wars*. London: Vintage Books, 2009.

Ramsey, J.H.R. 'A King, a Doctor and a Convenient Death' *British Medical Journal*, 308,6941 (1994) 1445.

Rose, S.O. *Which People's War? National Identity and Citizenship in Wartime Britain 1939–45*. Oxford: Oxford University Press, 2003.

Ross, C. *Twenties London: A City in the Jazz Age*. London: Philip Wilson, 2003.

Sandbrook, D. *Never Had It So Good: A History of Britain from Suez to the Beatles*. London: Brown, Little, 2006.

Savage, J. *Teenage: The Creation of Youth 1875–1945*. London: Pimlico, 2008.

Schenkar, J. *Truly Wilde: The Unsettling Story of Dolly Wilde, Oscar's Unusual Niece*. London: Virago, 2000.

Schlor, J. *Nights in the Big City: Paris, Berlin, London 1840–1930*. New York: Reaktion, 1998.

Schneider, E.C. *Smack: Heroin and the American City*. Philadelphia: University of Pennsylvania Press, 2008.

Schur, E.M. *Narcotic Addiction in Britain and America: The Impact of Public Policy*. London: Tavistock, 1963.

Seddon, T. *A History of Drugs: Drugs and Freedom in the Liberal Age*. Abingdon: Routledge, 2010.

Slater, S. 'Pimps, Police and Filles de Joie: Foreign Prostitution in Interwar London' *The London Journal*, 32,1 (2007) 53–74.

Smart, C. 'Social Policy and Drug Addiction: A Critical Study of Policy Development' *British Journal of Addiction* 79, (1984) 31–39.

Smart, C. 'Social Policy and Drug Dependence: An Historical Case Study' Drug *and Alcohol Dependence* 16 (1985) 169–180.

Spear, H.B. 'The Growth of Heroin Addiction in the United Kingdom' *British Journal of Addiction* 64, (1969) 245–255.

Spear, H.B. 'Conversation with H.B. Spear: Journal interview 20' *British Journal of Addiction*, 83, (1988) 473–482.

Spear, H.B. & Mott, J. 'Cocaine and Crack within the 'British System': A History of Control' in Bean, Philip, (ed.) *Cocaine and Crack: Supply and Use*. New York: St Martin's Press, 1993.

Spear, H.B. & (ed.) Mott, J. *Heroin Addiction, Care and Control: The British System*. London: Drugscope, 2002.
Spear, H.B. 'The early years of Britain's drug situation in practice: up to the 1960s' in Strang, J. & Gossop, M. (eds.) *Heroin Addiction and the British System: Volume 1*. London and New York: Routledge, 2005.
Steegmuller, F. *Cocteau: A Biography*. London: Constable, 1986.
Stevenson, J. *Edward Burra: Twentieth-Century Eye*. London: Pimlico, 2008.
Stimson, G. & Oppenheimer, E. *Heroin Addiction: Treatment and Control in Britain*. London: Tavistock, 1982.
Strang, J. & Gossop, M. (eds.) *Heroin Addiction and the British System: Origins and Evolution*. Abingdon: Routledge, 2005.
Summerscale, K. *The Queen of Whale Cay*. London: Fourth Estate, 1997.
Swanson, G. *Drunk with the Glitter: Space, consumption and sexual instability in modern urban culture*. Abingdon & New York: Routledge, 2007.
Sweet, M. *Shepperton Babylon: The Lost Worlds of British Cinema*. London: Faber and Faber, 2006.
Sweet, M. *West End Front: The Wartime Secrets of London's Grand Hotels*. London: Faber and Faber, 2011.
Tate, B. *West End Girls: The real lives, loves and friendship of 1940s Soho and its working girls*. London: Orion Books, 2010.
Taylor, D.J. *Bright Young People The Rise and Fall of a Generation: 1918–1940*. London: Chatto and Windus, 2007.
Thane, P. 'Population Politics in Post-War British Culture' in Conekin, Becky, Mort, Frank & Waters, Chris (eds.) (1999) *Moments of Modernity: Reconstructing Britain 1945–1964*. London & New York: Rivers Oram Press, 114–133.
Tinkler, P. *Smoke Signals: Women, smoking and visual culture*. Oxford: Berg, 2006.
Trebach, A.S. *The Heroin Solution, Second Edition*. Bloomington, Indiana: Unlimited Publishing, 2006.
Tripp, M. 'Who Speaks for Petro?' *Drugs and Society*, 3, (1973) 12–17
United Nations Office on Drugs and Crime. *A Century of International Drug Control*. Vienna: United Nations, 2009.
Vanderbilt, A. *The Best-Kept Boy in the World* New York City: Riverdale Avenue Books, 2014.
Walkowitz, J.R. *Nights Out: Life in Cosmopolitan London*. New Haven & London: Yale University Press, 2012.
Webber, J. 'Existentialism' in J. Skorupski (ed.), *Routledge Companion to Ethics*. London: Routledge, 2012.
Weinberger, B. *The Best Police in the World: An Oral History of English Policing from the 1930s to the 1960s*. Aldershot: Scolar Press, 1995.
White, J. *London in the 20th Century*. London: Vintage Books, 2008.
Whynes, D.K. & Bean, P. *Policing and Prescribing: The British System of Drug Control*. Basingstoke: Macmillan, 1991.

Wilson, E. *Bohemians: The Glamorous Outcasts.* London: Tauris Parke, 2003.
Young, J. *The Drugtakers: the Social Meaning of Drug Use.* London: MacGibbon & Kee, 1971.
Young, J. *The Vertigo of late Modernity.* London: Sage publications, 2007.
Zieger, S. *Inventing the Addict: Drugs, Race and Sexuality in Nineteenth Century British and American Literature.* Amherst: University of Massachusetts, 2008.
Ziegler, P. *Dianna Cooper.* London: Hamish Hamilton, 1981.

Unpublished Sources

Crossen White, H.L. *Drug related activity in the United Kingdom of Great Britain and Ireland between 1900 and 1922: What evidence can be found through systematic searches of The Times Digital Archive?* Unpublished PhD Thesis, Bournemouth, 2012.
Edwards, B. *Making the West End Modern: Space, Architecture and Shopping in 1930s London.* Unpublished PhD Thesis. London: University of the Arts, 2004.
Mars, S. *Prescribing and Proscribing: The Public-Private relationship in the treatment of Drug Addiction in England, 1970–99.* Unpublished PhD Thesis, University of London, 2006.
Slater, S. *Street sex for sale in Soho 1918–39: Experiences, Representation and Attempts at Control.* Unpublished PhD Thesis, University of London, 2007.

Websites

British modern jazz: From the 1940s onwards http://henrybebop.co.uk/bebop.htm
Cocktails with Elvira: Elvira Barney and her circle https://elvirabarney.wordpress.com/category/case-history/

Tate Website

Stephenson, A. '*New Ways of Modern Bohemia': Edward Burra in London, Paris, Marseilles and Harlem* Tate Papers Issue 1919 (2013). http://www.tate.org.uk/research/publications/tate-papers/new-ways-modern-bohemia-edward-burra-london-paris-marseilles-and Accessed 23 March 2015

Live Music Exchange

Williamson, J. *From the Musicians' Union Archive: Archer Street* http://livemusic-exchange.org/blog/from-the-musicians-union-archive-archer-street-john-williamson/
Dublin Institute of Technology http://arrow.dit.ie/aaconmusart/4/

Index[1]

[1] Note: Page numbers followed by 'n' refer to notes.

C. Hallam, *White Drug Cultures and Regulation in London, 1916–1960*, https://doi.org/10.1007/978-3-319-94770-9

FSC
www.fsc.org
MIX
Papier | Fördert
gute Waldnutzung
FSC® C083411

Kolibri 360 GmbH
Ferdinand-Jühlke-Straße 7
99095 Erfurt, Deutschland
produktsicherheit@kolibri360.de